The Doctor's Ultimate Guide to Contracts & Negotiations

Power Moves™!

Bonnie Simpson Mason, MD

Printed in the United States of America
ISBN: 9781513658834

Not intended as legal advice. For educational purposes only.

DEDICATION

This book is dedicated to my current/future physician colleagues, especially those on the front lines of COVID-19.

ACKNOWLEDGEMENTS

My first thanks go to God for tethering me to this gift through its completion against my best efforts to not do so, as humans so often do.

Of course, my husband and Bear Cubs have been rooting me on, while exercising tremendous patience, throughout this journey. Words can never express my love for my 3 Bears from Chicago.

Then, there is my lifelong core rooted in my mother's wisdom, my sister's encouragement and late night shoulder, my dad's spiritual boosts. I have experienced indescribable support from these three people thought my entire life for which I am eternally grateful. This level of love has been extended to me from my entire family, from the Simpsons and Youngs to the Pearsons and Masons.

For me, family has never been defined solely by genetics. I reflect on the expanse of my family and friends from East Point, GA to Howard University, from Morehouse School of Medicine to Mocha Medicine and Medical Moguls, from the HoCo Ladies to the Good Wives, from Nth Dimensions to Beyond the Exam Room and more. My gratitude is endless to all, especially to my orthopaedic surgery sisters and brothers.

Then to everyone who has trusted me as your mentor, Coach, educator and sounding board, what a privilege to be trusted in the ways. Then, to be able to call on friends and colleagues, Dr. Lauren Powell, Dr. Nicole Redmond, Dr. Lisa Whitty Bradley, Dr. Roseanne Gichuru, Dr. Ashley Mallory and Dr. Mom herself to preliminary review and edit this work means the world to me.

I cannot forget the expertise of Linda Engram, from Elly Virtually, in bringing this project to fruition with gentle nudges of support, and to the Pinnacle Conference Leadership and colleagues who were my first purchasers who have patiently waited for this to come to fruition, thank you.

In the end, I would like to thank my mentors/friends, Dr. Richard E. Grant, Dr. J. Mandume Kerina, Dr. Patricia Turner, Dr. Ronald Baker, Dr. Yolanda Wimberly, Verona Brewton, Tonya Primus, Ebony Halliburton and Kathryn O'Brien, who have believed in my vision for this work. Specifically, I deeply appreciate my coaches, Dr. Larthenia Howard, Dr. Draion Burch, Mikki Williams and my legal advisor/ coach, Attorney Randi Kopf.

Indeed, it takes a village, and I am eternally grateful for mine.

TESTIMONIALS

Dr. Simpson Mason has taken decades of experience, exceptional skill and merged it with her captivating personality to make a 'Must Read' manual for every medical professional-those just venturing out into practice, as well as those who may be reassessing their journey or renegotiating an established contract. When I had no choice but to start reviewing and negotiating my professional contracts, I was looking for a smart, concise, approachable and insightful manual to approach contract negotiation. This. Is. That. Guide.

Lisa Whitty Bradley, MD FACS – Plastic Surgeon, Author

I really appreciate Dr Mason for creating a very valuable resource that has been tremendously helpful and elucidating. As a recent Family Medicine resident transitioning as a practicing attending, this book was right on time! Her book is so comprehensive unlike articles I've read trying to put information together to learn about contracts and negotiations from a medical-legal perspective. The wealth of information she provided in this book was very easy to understand and digest, not to mention her style of writing made the content interesting! I think of it as a "Contract & Negotiations for Dummies" book with personality!

After being led by Dr Bonnie and incorporating what she taught me before and after signing my contract, I felt like I did my due diligence to feel comfortable and happy with my decision to work at my current place of employment. I also know that her book has made a significantly positive impact on improving my financial portfolio. If you are a graduating resident or seasoned physician looking to protect your mental well-being, family, profession, and finances before signing, updating, or resigning out of a contract, you'll definitely want to get this book!"

Ashley Mallory, MD – Family Medicine

After completing my BTER Elite Coaching Sessions with Dr. Bonnie, I was able to negotiate for a total compensation package that was 40% higher than my current package! Thank you, Dr. Bonnie, for giving me the tools, resources and confidence to negotiate for my true value as an employed physician. ALL doctors need to invest in ourselves and our futures by taking this course. Thank you again!

Monique Gary, DO, MSc, FACS - Breast Surgical Oncologist, Medical Director

I took Dr. Bonnie's contract catalyst course b/c I was trying to negotiate an issue I had at work regarding creating another business. The course helped me have the confidence to have the appropriate critical conversations with my partners and as a result was able to clear the air at my office regarding my business new business.

She gave a wealth of valuable info and I also took what I learned in the course to negotiate another contract and was able to $25k more b/c of asking some simple questions. I'm forever grateful to Dr. Bonnie and would recommend her course to anyone in medicine who has a contract! Thank you, Dr. Bonnie!

Brad Bellard, MD – Emergency Medicine, High Performance Coach

I have had the honor and pleasure to work with Dr. Bonnie Mason during my first few years as an attending. Her advice and guidance with navigating being a new physician, establishing relationships with the important people, and integrating my work life with my home life have been invaluable. Dr. Mason helped me to develop a system at work so that I am able to accurately record my productivity so that I have my own data when going to meetings with my supervisor. Dr. Mason has worked with many physicians, I call her The Physician's Mentor! I'm so glad to have her in my corner and know that my career would be in a different place right now without her.

Lauren Powell, MD – Family Medicine, The Culinary Doctor

I would like to thank Dr. Bonnie for her expertise in assisting me to negotiate my Medical Director agreement for my hospital system.

Dr. Bonnie taught me strategy, ways to effectively communicate with administration and also gave a referral to legal counsel, which was paramount in achieving successful negotiations. Previously, I have had experience with contract negotiations and felt confident. However, I wish I took this course sooner because I now realize my past negotiations mistakes. Without the course, I don't think I would have been able to negotiate a 100% increase in my eligible income. I highly recommend Dr. Bonnie's contract catalyst course to anyone engaging in Contract Negotiations.

Roland Hamilton, MD – Neurology, Medical Director

I sought out Dr. Bonnie as I was preparing to transition out of my current OB-GYN practice. Over the past several months, I had done the work of identifying my options, and the benefits and trade-off associated with each option. There was a lot of uncertainty and numerous moving parts that caused me a lot of anxiety. I knew I needed another set of eyes to assist me with making the right decision.
Enter Dr. Bonnie.

She listened and challenged me in the oddest of ways; from questioning some of my decisions to asking seemingly random questions. We laugh about it now but looking back she was encouraging me to bring more of "me" to the decision-making process. Dr. Bonnie looked at my scenario and recognized that it was missing my "other goals". I had addressed my career pursuits but inadvertently left out my life goals. She helped me bring "me" to my career goals. Thank you, Dr. Bonnie!

Roseanne Gichuru, DO – Obstetrics and Gynecology

"Dr. Bonnie understands that the physician model of education and training is NOT well-suited to negotiating with business executives, who have been at this game since their early 20s. Dr. Bonnie employs a philosophy of "Think Like a Business Person, Not a Physician" so that we are in a position to begin taking medicine and healthcare from the hands of corporations--for ourselves and for our communities. "

Andrea M. Brownridge, MD JD MHA - Psychiatry

"Dr. Bonnie is an amazing and phenomenal physician to have as a mentor. It was through her program that I not only learned about myself but that I was also able to take that knowledge and use it to express those wants and needs in a way that was adequately reflected in my contract. I learned that the expression of those essentials is not optional, and that this expression is what adds to a balanced work-life integration. I truly found my voice with Dr. Bonnie and I will be forever grateful."

Shani Smith, DO, MBA – Critical Care Medicine

Dr. Bonnie, I cannot thank you enough. I cannot thank you enough for all of your support and insight during a very difficult time in my practice. Yes, I had a lawyer, but I truly benefited from having the voice and insight of an experienced physician who helped me navigate the necessary steps that I needed to take, calmed me down, and believed that I could actually win in what I thought was a losing situation. Thank you so much!

Jovan Adams, DO – Family Medicine

DISCLAIMER

The information provided in this book does not, and is not intended to, constitute legal advice; instead, all information, content, and materials available on this site are for general informational purposes only. Information in this book may not constitute the most up-to-date legal or other information. This book contains references and links to other third-party websites. Such references and links are only for the convenience of the reader, user or browser.

Readers of this book should contact their attorney to obtain advice with respect to any particular legal matter. No reader or user of this book should act or refrain from acting on the basis of information in this book without first seeking legal advice from counsel in the relevant jurisdiction. Only your individual attorney can provide assurances that the information contained herein – and your interpretation of it – is applicable or appropriate to your particular situation. Use of, and access to, this book or any of the links or resources contained within the book do not create an attorney-client relationship between the reader, user, or browser and website authors, contributors, contributing law firms, or committee members and their respective employers.

The views expressed at, or through, this book are those of the individual author writing in the author's individual capacities only – not those of the author's respective employer, association or committee/task force with which the author may be affiliated as a whole. All liability with respect to actions taken or not taken based on the contents of this book is hereby expressly disclaimed. The content in this book is provided "as is;" no representations are made that the content is error-free.

TABLE OF CONTENTS

Not intended as legal advice. For educational purposes only.

SECTION 3 - MASTERING OUR NEGOTIATIONS

SECTION 4 - THE APPENDICES

Introduction

"Doctors are in healthcare. Healthcare is a business. Therefore, doctors are in business."

~Dr. Bonnie Simpson Mason

I know this may be disheartening, disappointing, and frustrating to us doctors, but this is our new reality, and the sooner we accept this and get in the game by learning about business, the better. How do we do this? By starting with learning the essential fundamentals of business, more specifically, contracts, which we were not taught in medical school or in training. I am convinced that advocating for ourselves beginning with our contracts is the #1 way that we can protect ourselves and get paid our worth.

I affirm that we can digest this new language and evolve into the leaders that are needed to protect patients, our families, and ourselves while practicing medicine in the 21st century.

Who am I?

I am Bonnie Simpson Mason, MD, who in the midst of learning to run a small private orthopedic surgery practice and becoming board-certified in orthopedic surgery, retired early due to disability secondary to rheumatoid arthritis. Ultimately, I had to retire permanently from practicing medicine in my early thirties, but only after learning the hard way that we as doctors are in no way trained or equipped to navigate either the business, financial or the contractual aspects of practicing medicine.

I am not a lawyer, but I have conferred and partnered with health law attorneys consistently over the years to understand contracts while serving as the physician educator in my own practice. So, I know firsthand the level of stress, inadequacy, and uncertainty that we as doctors can feel when faced with making business, contractual, financial, human resource, legal, accounting, and strategic decisions without having a sound foundation.

In short, I found my frustration mounting while being forced to make these non-clinical, but critical business and practice decisions day after day with absolutely no education or training on how to do so. Then, I decided to take action, and I joined forces with another board-certified physician to develop Beyond the Exam Room, a curriculum on healthcare economics and the business of medicine for residents and fellows. What began as a textbook, which we did not publish, has morphed into live sessions, online modules, webinars, and masterclasses for hundreds of physicians annually since we began this work in 2004.

Over the past 20 years, I have had the opportunity to educate thousands, mentored hundreds and serve as a career strategist and contracts coach for doctors in practice and in training across the country through my educational firm, Beyond the Exam Room, and via my philanthropic work having founded the non-profit organization, Nth Dimensions.

Why I wrote this book?

In recent years, the distress calls I have received from doctor-colleagues have been unfortunate, heartbreaking and, in some cases, unconscionable,
such as:

- o   They won't like me if I negotiate.
- o   I am working so hard, sometimes with no lunch and no time to even go to the bathroom. Yet, I am being told that I am not covering my overhead.
- o   I need to move because of family reasons, but I can't afford to leave.
- o   I've been at this practice for 12 years, and I've never received a raise, nor have I renegotiated my contract.
- o   I was just told that my salary is being decreased by $100K next year.
- o   I am being terminated in 30 days, they say without cause, but I don't know what that means.
- o   I am being treated so poorly. I need to leave, but I am so afraid.
- o   I have been on call every other day for 54 weeks straight. I have no choice but to leave this practice.
- o   I am watching unscrupulous care being delivered as dictated by the leadership here. I do not want to lose my license. What do I do?

Unfortunately, there is a common thread integrating among all of these sentiments:

- o Fear of the impact on their career and personal life
- o Disappointment in the fact that after all of the years of sacrifice, someone is making a business-based decision, despite the excellent level of care provided
- o Lack of knowledge about their contractual rights, options, and opportunities to address each of the above through advocating via critical conversations, i.e., via negotiations

However, I am happy to report that close to 100% of the doctors I've worked with to address these situations have #won! For that, I have been given the nickname of *The Olivia Pope for Doctors*, which I think is a great thing.

Winning in these situations, many of which have been borne out of the corporatization of the entire healthcare system, has required hours of educating, strategizing, and informal coaching in partnership with these doctors.

Who is this book for?

Due to the current trends in the physician workforce moving more physicians towards becoming employees after completing their training, this book is for you or someone you know if you are:

- o A doctor in training and in the midst of searching for your initial clinical job, and the thought of signing your first employment contract without a clue scares you to death (it should)
- o A practicing doctor transitioning to your next position, and you don't want to sign another contract blindly (like you did the first time)
- o A clinician with a doctorate who is entering or transitioning into practice (because these employment contracts closely parallel those of physicians)

- o Have a friend, colleague, or family member who is a resident, fellow or young doctor in practice, and you want to be supportive (friends don't let friends sign contracts without a clue)
- o A medical educator at any level and are looking for a resource to provide your trainees with information to assist them with their transition into the real world

While this book is aimed at educating younger doctors who are within 5 years of completing training, I would anticipate that seasoned doctors might also use this book as a resource to answer specific contract and negotiation questions as well.

How to use this book:

This book parallels our basic science years in medical school by laying the foundational knowledge about the core contract and negotiation concepts, as explained by one doctor to another.

- o Section 1 challenges us to stop, be introspective, and be empowered through changing our mindsets and taking requisite actions.
- o Section 2 then delves into the core components of an employment contract.
- o We end with Section 3, which reveals the key negotiation strategies I found myself using with countless numbers of docs, which I hope will help you, as well.

I chose to start with creating a guide to contracts and negotiations because this subject tends to be the most requested lecture content, Master Class content, and webinar content.

Each chapter ends with a Chapter Summary, which includes:

Power Moves – These are my Dr. Bonnie's Pearls, lessons learned personally and those that I have shared with doctors. (See Appendix A for my Playbook of Power Moves)

Take-Home Points – Key takeaways of the most important concepts from each chapter

Red Flags – Landmines and points of caution that I want us to avoid

Homework – Follow-up actionable steps highlighted to help us achieve the goals in each chapter

Finally, please observe the following intentions:

What this book is:

- o Easy to read vs. labor intensive.
- o Digestible with the intentional, anatomical, and clinical references.
- o Fundamentally sound referencing of Black's Law Library, one of the most commonly accepted reference dictionaries for attorneys.
- o Based on hundreds of doctor encounters, challenges, and experiences
- o A resource written FOR DOCTORS BY DOCTORS to help us become better-informed clients when working with our health law attorney, in the same way, that we as doctors engage better with informed patients.

What this book is NOT:

- o A substitute for retaining a health law attorney. #Getalawyer!
- o A legal reference by proxy

I wrote this book to fill the educational void in our medical education system that ensures that we are clinically adept at rendering excellent care to our patients but has failed to prepare us on how to navigate in the real world of practicing in the 21st century. It is my goal to share many of the tools, roadmaps, as well as some proven doctor-to-doctor strategies to steer us for the win.

I've been and remain blessed to serve in this role, provide hope and encouragement, build awareness, and educate my colleagues in this arena. The reward has been hearing the level of relief on the other end from doctors who have moved from:

o   tears to joy
o   nervous to knowledgeable
o   uninformed and unaware to empowered advocates for themselves

We can do this, Docs! We absolutely can do this.

To this end, I hope this book serves you well and that you will share one with one of your doctor colleagues, residents, or students as well.

At the end of the day, one thing I know for sure is that when we are better informed, we make better decisions and live our best lives.

Let's learn the business and financial sides of medicine, starting now!

Chapter 1

START WITH WHY

~Simon Sinek

Doc: *Dr. Bonnie, I don't know what happened. When I was going through my training, the local hospital said that they really wanted me to work there once I finished my training. I*
was just so happy that they liked me, that I signed the contract quickly, and I went straight to work upon graduation. Now, nothing is like I thought it would be. (This Doc was in tears at this point in the conversation.)

Dr. Bonnie: *I hear this so often. Doc, you are not alone. We just did not learn how to successfully transition into the real world in school or training. Lets start now by understanding why we are in this position and what we can do about it.*

I can't begin to count the number of times that I've heard the aforementioned scenario from doctors across the country.

There are so many reasons why this scenario plays out to the detriment of doctors, and we will cover these reasons in this chapter, namely:

o   Reviewing the big picture
o   The most important thing to remember about every contract you receive
o   The three most important Power Moves that we can make

The Big Picture

Well, I've said this in the introduction, and I will say it again,

> "Doctors are in healthcare.
> Healthcare is a business.
> Therefore, doctors are in business."

So, we must get in this mindset or remain victims of the decisions being made on our behalf by administrators who have not seen patients or who do not value the doctor-patient relationship. We can no longer claim that we are too busy seeing patients to become more knowledgeable, pay attention, or advocate for ourselves and our colleagues in the hospital, community, local or regional meetings where decisions are being made that affect our lives, our families, and our patients.

> In the legal field, ignorance is not a defense.
> In medicine, being busy is not an excuse.

Not convinced. Well, here are some facts about the US healthcare system as they relate to us doctors, the primary revenue generators in this system[1,2]:

o   Each doctor generates on average 7-8 figures of gross revenue for the hospital or medical center with which they are affiliated

- o The ratio of healthcare administrators to doctors is now 10:1
- o The cost to doctors who sign unfavorable contracts can amount to over $100,000, based on anecdotal evidence gathered from the hundreds of doctors that I have coached over the past 15 years.

Unquestionably, with the external healthcare environment becoming more tumultuous due to corporatization, doctors must take control of the aspects of healthcare that are within our control. And certainly, understanding our contracts represents one major opportunity for us as individuals to negotiate our worth and educate the 20,000 new doctors that we launch into practice annually. Educating our current and future doctor colleagues represents the responsibility we have as current doctors to ensure the professional and personal well-being of those coming behind us.

What the Employment Contract Represents to Doctors

OUR EMPLOYMENT CONTRACT IS THE SINGLE MOST IMPORTANT DOCUMENT THAT WE WILL SIGN, BECAUSE IT:

- o Dictates our professional lives and, by default, our personal lives, as well.
  - o More specifically, it details how your time will be spent clinically, administratively, educationally which affects how much personal time will be left.
- o Serves as a vehicle to protect us as we practice medicine in one of the most litigious industries in the US
- o Details the complex models by which we will be compensated

Top 3 Proactive Power Moves Doctors Can Make

The most important thing about contracts that everyone needs to digest and remember:

> **Power Move #1** - *ALWAYS REMEMBER that contracts are written in favor of the AUTHOR of the contract!*

In this context, the author of the contract is the employer, who hires legal counsel to draft a contract that will encompass ALL of the employer's terms and stipulations.

Though it's not unreasonable to think that the hospital/practice will include contract terms that work in our favor, my point is that it is not the employer's responsibility to do so. It is our responsibility to learn how to analyze our contracts, advocate for ourselves, and negotiate on our own behalf.

This is the primary concept that I want to drive home, especially for our younger physicians, along with the following:

- o We should never assume that our needs (and wants) are reflected in ANY contract we receive.
- o We MUST retain our own health law attorney, who will partner with us to ensure that our needs and wants are reflected in the contract. The employer's attorney is NOT and cannot serve as our attorney, simultaneously.

> **Power Move #2** - *Give yourself the gift of time during your job search!*

Each of us can attest to the relationship between time and stress, which I dare say in contracts and negotiations are inversely proportional.

Remember when we could cram for an exam in undergraduate school and could likely squeeze through with an acceptable grade? However, in medical school, we found out VERY quickly that ample time was needed in order to digest the volume of material that we needed to digest quickly. We found that the more time we gave ourselves to study for exams, especially for boards, that our anxiety decreased somewhat. Conversely, when we did not commit the time, then our stress and anxiety became virtually unbearable.

More time → Less stress

Less time → More stress

This is the first step to integrating an "informed decision-making" process into our professional and personal lives, not just our clinical decisions. We must apply the same rigor, standards, and data requirements for the decisions that we make beyond the exam room. Indeed, we want to work smarter, not harder, and by all means, I want you to avoid making the same mistakes that myself and so many other seasoned doctors have made regarding business, contractual and financial decisions.

Remember when we applied to medical school during the summer before our senior year in college? Similarly, we began researching desired residency programs approximately a year or so before the Match.

See, we've done this before, so let's apply the same time frame and approach to the process of transitioning into our first (or next) position as a practicing doctor as well.

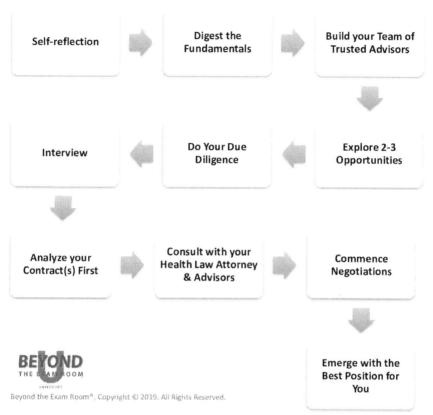

Figure 1 – The 10-Step Contract and Negotiations Process

I wanted to provide an overview of the process required to transition into our first or next position strategically and with intention. Figure 1 depicts The 10-Step Contract and Negotiations Process that I recommend my fellow doctors use as a transitional guide. (See Appendix B)

Moreover, I must caution you, my fellow doctor colleagues, that signing your employment contract is the culmination of what should be an 18-24 month strategically planned out search and fact-finding process aimed at transitioning you into your first or next position as an employed doctor as successfully as possible. However, we must first employ due diligence.

Power Move #3 - *We must do our due diligence!*

Due diligence is a legal term that I want all doctors to become familiar with, especially as it pertains to how we should regard any contract that we are reviewing.

As defined by Black's Law Dictionary, due diligence refers to exercising:

o   prudence - acting with or showing care and thought about the future
o   assiduity - constant or close attention to what one is doing as is properly to be expected from, and ordinarily exercised by a reasonable and prudent man under the particular circumstances.

I love that this definition of due diligence highlights activities that show care, as well as thoughtful and close attention to what we are doing, in our case with regards to our contracts.

More specifically, doing our due diligence regarding our contracts can be defined as taking time to:

o   analyze our contracts for ourselves
o   understand practice trends in our specialty
o   research our respective fair market values for compensation
o   patient and practice demographics for our desired practice types
o   engage in meaningful discussions with our health law attorney and other advisors

Performing this level of research and investigation about our specialty and practice, as reflected in our contracts, will undoubtedly require a considerable amount of time, and these are yet additional reasons why the 18-24 month transition time frame is suggested.

More importantly, doing our due diligence will allow us to acquire the information we need to use "informed decision-making" when making critical contract, business, and financial decisions.

So, moving forward, let's please do our due diligence, i.e., educating ourselves, doing our research, securing input from trusted advisors, and negotiating our worth before signing ANY contract in the future.

> ## *Power Move #4* - *SIP to Success Strategy™*

I want to end this chapter with an original framework that I developed to help us as physicians adjust our mindsets when it comes to how we think about matters beyond the exam room. Although we have been strategically planning our entire medical career throughout our lives, I want to talk to you about applying those same principles to the non-clinical aspects of our lives.

I want us to SIP our way to success. By implementing my *SIP to Success Strategy™*, I want us to strategically think about being intentional with our documentation and proactive with our communication with the decision-makers both at work and at home.

- o **S** is for being purposefully STRATEGIC
- o **I** is for being INTENTIONAL about out documenting our strategy, and
- o **P** is for being PROACTIVE about communicating with our supervisors, our healthcare team, and our practice administrators

We must assert ourselves in today's healthcare environment by thinking strategically and by taking a proactive approach to having a successful career.

This approach is in contrast to how we are trained to function clinically. We are taught how to react when encountering running a code or when operating on abnormal anatomy. Even more, we prepare ourselves to react evenly with every patient that we encounter behind the next exam room door or emergency room curtain. However, this reactive conditioning and mindset does not serve us well in the world of contracts, hence my recommendation to use the *SIP to Success Strategy™* as often as possible.

True story: I remember sharing the *SIP to Success Strategy™* approach with a young physician who had been in practice for just under one year. Her administrator was already letting her know that at the end of her first year in which she had a guaranteed salary that her salary would be decreased by 20% in her second year of practice. I recommended that the doctor start thinking strategically by:

- o review her contract to clarify the number of Relative Value Units (to be discussed in detail in chapter 9) required - *Strategic*
- o analyzing the efficiency of her workflow - *Strategic*
- o documenting her productivity with intention on a routine, weekly basis - Intentional Documentation
- o proactively scheduling monthly meetings with her administrator to review her productivity and the subsequent calculation of her RVUs - Proactive communication

Upon doing so, the doctor was able to resolve scheduling and workflow challenges within the office that were impacting her productivity. She was also able to verify whether the practice's documentation of her productivity correlated with the actual numbers of patients that she was seeing (or not). As a result, she was subsequently able to maintain her salary without any decrease in pay. She also developed stronger relationships with her administrators by taking an interest in the sustainability of the practice overall.

By using the *SIP to Success Strategy™,* I want us to think about being intentional with our documentation and proactive with our communication with the decision-makers, both at home and at work. When we employ a strategy, then we are leaving very few things to chance. We are planning out and setting some specific milestones and benchmarks for ourselves that we want to meet so that we can live the lives we want to lead.

The SIP to Success Strategy™ can also be applied to our personal lives, as well.

Just as we spent years studying to become doctors who are prepared to autonomously care for patients, we must take ample time to prepare to transition into the career that we wish to have.

Suffice it to say, gaining an understanding of contracts and becoming a confident negotiator and advocate require an ongoing commitment to learning about and conferring with others on this subject.

CHAPTER SUMMARY

POWER MOVES

- o Remember that contracts are written in favor of the author of the contract
- o Give ourselves the gift of time when embarking on the journey to find our first or next position
- o We must do our due diligence in researching potential positions and subsequently reviewing our contracts
- o Apply the *SIP to Success Strategy™* to both our professional and personal lives

TAKE-HOME POINTS

Digesting, mastering, and conquering our contracts are achievable goals if we take the following steps:

- o Begin learning about contracts at least 18-24 months prior to signing our first employment agreement. This is the same lead-time that we took to apply to medical school and residency. We should allow ourselves the same time to prepare to transition into our first or next practice.
- o Do our due diligence so that we can apply an "informed decision-making" process to our career and our contract negotiations.

HOMEWORK

- o As adult learners, we require repetition, rigor, and relevance. Continue learning about contracts and the business/financial aspects of medicine on a routine, ongoing basis.

REFERENCES

1. Miller, P. New Survey Shows Physicians Are Key Revenue Generators for Hospitals. https://www.merritthawkins.com/news-and-insights/blog/healthcare-news-and-trends/new-survey-shows-physicians-are-key-revenue-generators-for-hospitals/

2. Kocher, R. The Downside of Health Care Job Growth. https://hbr.org/2013/09/the-downside-of-health-care-job-growth.

NOTES

Chapter 2

PHYSICIAN KNOW THYSELF (& YOUR WORTH)

Doc: *I think that I'm making a decent salary, but I am on call so often that I don't have time to care for my aging parents nor to have a life. This is not working for me and my family.*

Dr. Bonnie: *I totally understand. Yes, there is so much more than one salary that should be considered when accepting a new position. Understanding our needs and wants is critical to helping us build the professional and personal lives than we desire and deserve.*

For many of us, our goal in becoming a doctor was to achieve a fulfilled life while caring for patients. We knew that achieving this would require relentless dedication, arduous studying, delayed gratification, and sacrifices beyond measure from us as individuals.

In order to achieve this fulfilled life, both professionally and personally, it is up to us to define our core values along with our specific needs and requirements that will help us achieve this goal. Unfortunately, this is an exercise that most doctors have not been encouraged to reflect upon before signing our first, second or third contract. Instead we have primarily conditioned to put our needs aside for the benefit of our profession and patients, while often sacrificing our own well-being, and subsequently that of our families. Wow! What price to pay.

Therefore, I strongly suggest that as we transition into or between practices, it is our responsibility to take the time to identify our core values, our needs (and also our wants) in pursuit of this fulfilled life for the ultimate benefit of our families, our patients and ourselves.

Work-Life Integration

I refer to this intersection of our professional and personal lives using a work-life integration model, as described in the lay literature by authors such as Betz, Kimsey-House and Uhereczky. I reference the work-life integration framework primarily because I have observed both in my life and in the lives of the hundreds of doctors that I have mentored and coached that major career decisions ALWAYS affect both our work lives AND our personal lives, not just one or the other.

Personally, I reached this conclusion after years of being a doctor entrepreneur, especially when I realized that every work decision, I made also affected my life and my finances. Conversely, every decision I made at home influenced my practice or business. My husband is also a doctor, and I recognized the same patterns emerging in his life, as well. At no time have I found that I came close to reaching the illusive work-life balance position, to my dismay.

Instead, I observed more of an ongoing ebb and flow taking place in my life. At times, the focus of my attention seemed to ebb toward work as I studied for my orthopaedic surgery boards while simultaneously building a private practice. Then, the emphasis in my life flowed more towards my personal life once my children were born. For me, there was never an even 50/50 split of my attention to work and life, which proved to be frustrating and disappointing. I did not know what I was doing wrong.

Then, I chose to shift my mindset. When I truly began to embrace the ebb and flow nature of my career, business, financial, and personal decisions in an integrated fashion, I actually felt relieved. The relief stemmed from not having to make the dichotomous choice between work and life but learning that I could bend with the flow when work and life moved in one direction together, not in competition with one another.

Reframing my approach to one of embracing work-life integration subsequently impacted all of my relationships, both at work and at home. It gave me a framework to use when contemplating how my work commitments affected the decisions that needed to be made in my personal life. Here are some of examples of work-life integration questions that we can ask ourselves:

- o If I am starting a new practice/business in the late summer, which is also my vacation time, how can I adapt my vacation plans to free up more time to transition into practice?
- o March is a busy month for medical conferences, but my absence certainly affects my personal life. We will need some additional help with childcare, which will impact our budget. What financial steps can be taken in advance to fund these childcare needs for the month?

Notice, the aim is to always consider how my career/business decisions will affect my family and my finances, rather than looking at one independently of the other.

I also end these statements with a question to open the door for bi-directional communication with the other person being affected

26

by the changes in my career/life. (You can thank me later for these free #husband/wife/partner points.)

Check out this super cool Venn diagram below, which illustrates work-life integration graphically.

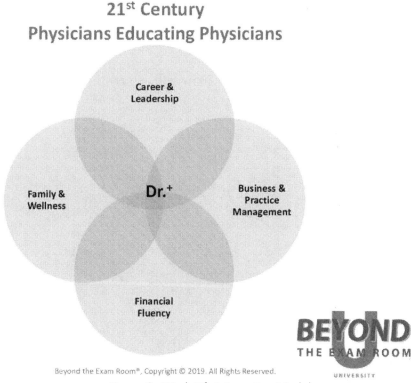

Beyond the Exam Room®, Copyright © 2019. All Rights Reserved.

Figure 2 - Work-Life Integration Model

That's us in the middle, the Doctor with an asterisk representing our accountability partner, whom we should enlist to help us navigate these unchartered waters in our lives.

Please observe that each circle, which represents different life commitments, overlaps and affects the other. Conversely, there is no way to make a career, business, financial or family decision that doesn't affect every other aspect of our lives.

For Educational Purposes Only. Not Intended as Legal Advice.

Once again, integrating this work-life integration concept has been liberating for me, and I no longer feel like I have to choose work OR life. I can actually choose both while understanding that this work-life integration model may lean more towards work at times, then towards personal life at others.

> ***Power Move #5*** *- Forget Work-Life Balance.*
> *Consider Work-Life Integration!*

The good news is that we don't have to make these decisions alone or in isolation, because we are in the center of this paradigm, along with our accountability partner (to be discussed in Chapter 3), whom we should work with to help us make both professional and personal decisions.

We can then recruit a team of trusted advisors who should also support our work-life integration approach to informed decision-making, leading us steps closer to living our best lives, one decision at a time.

DOCS, THE FOLLOWING SECTION MAY BE THE MOST IMPORTANT SECTION IN THIS ENTIRE BOOK!

Physician, Know Thyself First!

As Simon Sinek says, "Start with why."

Our individual needs and wants, including those of our family, are as specific to us as our fingerprints. No two doctors have the same personal, career or financial profiles. Because of the uniqueness of our situations, we should identify our needs and wants, starting with identifying our core values first. Then, we must negotiate to have these requirements for a fulfilled life incorporated into the document that governs our professional lives, which is our employment agreement.

Our employment agreement also governs our personal lives by default because it indirectly dictates how much time we will have to build a personal life after satisfying our professional commitments and obligations.

This is where the overlap and intersection of our professional and personal occurs, and this is why it is imperative that we negotiate in order to live the life we want and deserve.

> *Power Move #6* - *Doctors, we must know our needs and our wants, because WE matter!*

First, here are a set of reflection exercises that I recommend every doctor discover or rediscover before moving into contract negotiations:

1. Our core values, which should ideally align with those of our employer
2. Our needs and wants, which we will negotiate into our contract in order to protect ourselves and the things that are dear to us

Core Values

Let's think for a few minutes about what drives us as individuals, both professionally and personally.

Do honesty, love, and integrity characterize who you are at home and at work?

Are you committed to working as a team, being loyal, and displaying excellence at all times?

These are just some examples of core values. Understanding our core values can help us identify positions that may be a good fit, if the organization has a culture and core values that are similar to ours.

Some organizations emphasize inclusion and problem-solving amongst their healthcare providers. Others prioritize communication with and wellness for their physicians in order to achieve optimal patient care outcomes.

It is our job to first identify our own core values, so that we can better look for similar core values from our potential employers.

Check out Section 1 of your Power Moves Workbook and take a few minutes to contemplate then record your top 3 core values.

Let's Uncover our Needs and Wants

I think each of us can relate to the arduous, unrelenting nature of medical education at the undergraduate, medical school, and residency/fellowship training levels.

The stringent nature of training at every level has taught us to be outwardly focused and somewhat neglectful of ourselves, primarily because every clinical decision can mean life or death for one of our patients. We know this, and we know how this level of responsibility feels.

Yet while in the process of becoming fully immersed in the world of medical school, followed by the unrelenting pledging process of residency, we tend to lose sight of some of our needs and our wants.

Well, it's time for us to get back to the core of who we are and what drives us, so we can advocate and negotiate for a position that helps us return to the fullness of who we are.

So, I would like to encourage us to take a few moments to reflect on who we are today, and what our needs and wants are TODAY.

Why?

Because if we are unclear about what we truly need (which are our NON-NEGOTIABLES) and what we truly want (also known as

NEGOTIABLES), then we are limiting the possibilities of signing an employment agreement that creates a win-win for us and the other party.

- o Our NEEDS = NON-NEGOTIABLES, deal-breakers, must-haves
- o Our WANTS = NEGOTIABLES, nice to haves, can live with or without these (ideally with), icing on the cake

Doc, Your NEEDS Matter Most

In the process of securing your first or next position, it is absolutely CRITICAL that individual doctors determine for themselves what is truly important.

Just like the core needs of food, shelter, and water, which are identified in Maslow's Hierarchy of Needs[3], we, as adults on our individual paths, have developed needs and requirements in order to live our best lives.

Here are some examples. Perhaps, it is extremely important for you to:

- o Work in a particular location in order to care for your ailing parents
- o Find an academic position in order to continue your research
- o Not take overnight calls in-house because your spouse works at night
- o Pay off your student loans as quickly as possible
- o Be financially secure because you are the first doctor in your family, and they are depending on you
- o Walk your children to the bus stop in the morning in order to maximize the amount of time you can spend with them

The above represent types of *NEEDS,* accommodations, and requirements that you might deem absolutely necessary for you to achieve a certain quality of life.

Overall, your needs are non-negotiable! If your specific must-haves cannot be negotiated for in the process of finding your next position, then we have to be willing to walk away.

Yikes! Yes, I said that we must be willing to pursue other options if our needs cannot be met, and this is why your needs are also called deal-breakers.

Yes, we have worked for years in medical school and in training by sacrificing some of our needs, but we have to shift out of this mindset and work to achieve most if not all of our core needs moving forward.

> **Step 1** - Work with your accountability partner, colleague, or family member to begin developing a list of your needs and must-haves now.

> **Step 2** - Work with your health lawyer and physician mentor/coach to develop a strategy to integrate your needs into your contract.

As a result of identifying then integrating these needs into your contract negotiations, you will be able to perform maximally because your core needs have been met.

I continue to meet so many docs who did not negotiate their contracts at all. Initially, they were just happy to get a job, but they wound up being miserable because their core needs were not being met.

In doing so, they did not protect their own interests by negotiating with their employer ahead of time. As a result, these docs were working in a constant state of dissatisfaction, which led to stress, anxiety, and depression for many.

Nothing tears at my heart more than to hear a doctor in tears due to extreme distress, because they did not negotiate what they NEEDED into their contract. Now that you're reading this chapter, this no longer has to be the case.

(Remember, my esteemed colleagues, this is not residency. We do not have to settle for just any job or position. We want to find and negotiate for the best position for us.)

Your WANTS Also Matter

Your *wants* are important and represent the items that are nice to have, but you do not consider them an absolute deal-breaker if they are not negotiated into your contract. For example, perhaps you would like to have an additional week of paid time off (PTO) or leave? Is this a deal-breaker for you, or not?

You get to decide what is important for you, your career, and your life. Please note, that upon completing this self-reflection, reality dictates that *everything that is negotiable is negotiable*. So, is it likely that you will get everything that you need *and* want? I'm sure it's possible, but unlikely. However, if you are able to negotiate for your needs and a portion of your wants, you get to decide whether you will be happy or
satisfied with this.

Consider this comparison, your needs (non-negotiables) constitute the cake and the icing represents your wants (negotiables). Cake with no icing at least provides a strong foundation upon which future icing can be placed after future negotiations. However, icing with no cake is less desirable, because your foundation is not intact and your core need for cake has not been met. Right?

Also remember that contracts are strategically written by attorneys to include all of the wants, needs, and requirements that the employer or author deems necessary from their perspective.

It is neither the other party's responsibility nor obligation to include your wants and needs in any contract.

> *Power Move #7* - *It is always our responsibility to advocate for ourselves by asking and negotiating for what WE need and want.*

Time to Get to Work!

Now is your time to sit back and reflect on what you truly NEED and WANT at this particular point in your life, and this may take a little while since many of us put our own wants and needs on the back seat many years ago while in medical school or training. It's time to dig them up, and you may need to consult your accountability partner on this assignment.

For many of us, it is not as easy as one would think, so take as much time as you need.

This is important! Use the <u>Power Moves Needs and Wants Worksheet and Blueprint</u> in Section 1 of your Power Moves Workbook to complete this task. In the future, you will need to refer back to this list before and during your contract negotiations to provide clarity and self-confidence.

Your specific list of needs and wants should:

- o Reflect both personal and professional items
- o Prioritize your wants and needs from most to least important
- o Be as specific as possible

Power Moves Needs and Wants Blueprint - Here are some examples of actual needs and wants from physician colleagues.

Priority	Needs (Non-negotiables)	Priority	Wants (Negotiables)
1	To work in an outpatient setting; no weekend work hours	1	To be home by 5:30 p.m., 3-4 days/week to support my family's after school activities.
2	To have the employer pay for tail insurance.	2	To enroll for 10 additional online CMEs monthly
3	To be paid the fair market value hourly pay to be on call.	3	To the Bear Cubs 3-4 x per week before bed for 30 mins
4	To exercise 4 times per week before work.	4	To publish one peer-reviewed article in the next 6 months

Figure 3 - Power Moves Needs and Wants Blueprint

IMPORTANT: Identifying YOUR needs (non-negotiables) and wants (negotiables) is
THE MOST IMPORTANT EXERCISE
for you to complete BEFORE meeting with your health lawyer
and BEFORE entering into any contract negotiations.

Why? Because your needs are the terms that you need to ensure are negotiated into your contract BEFORE you sign, which provides you with security knowing that your needs are being met via your contract. No one can identify your negotiables, and more importantly your non-negotiables (your deal-breakers) for you, but you!

Doc: Isn't that what my attorney is for?

Dr. Bonnie: No, your health law attorney is retained to ensure that your contract legally binds you to the employment opportunity within the limits and legalities of the law as it pertains to healthcare.

Your health law attorney will ensure that the contract includes and reflects the terms that you deem as non-negotiable, IF you clearly communicate to the attorney what these critical components of your life are. Your Needs and Wants Blueprint will help to facilitate this conversation with your health law attorney, who is not a mind reader.

Just as we appreciate having an informed patient come to us for treatment because we can achieve a better health outcome in the doctor-patient relationship, our attorneys are best able to ensure that the contract reflects our wants and needs as well as being protective legally. Be an informed doctor-client!

Again, neither our health law attorneys nor any of our trusted advisors are mind readers. We must approach them with the clearest concepts about what we are looking for, and this is the self-reflection work and due diligence that each of us must do (with the help of our accountability partners) BEFORE transitioning into a new position.

As an additional resource, please refer to the <u>Power Moves Points of Negotiation</u> in Appendix C to review a list of additional points that physicians I have identified and negotiated for in the past. (Thank you to the Mocha Docs for your valued contributions to this list!

CHAPTER SUMMARY

POWER MOVES

- o Know your needs and your wants because YOU matter
- o Consider achieving work-life integration vs. work-life balance
- o We must advocate for our own needs and wants during contract negotiations, period.

TAKE-HOME POINTS

- o Work-life balance is a challenging construct. Consider embracing a Work-Life Integration paradigm.
- o Doc, you matter, as do your wants and needs.
- o Be as specific as possible when identifying your needs and wants
- o Know that your wants and needs will change over time (and they should).
- o In the future, revisit your Wants and Needs Blueprint before making any major life decisions to ensure that you stay in alignment with your true mission and ambitions.

RED FLAGS

- o Signing a contract without reflecting on your needs and wants can result in your new position satisfying the needs of the employer and not yours.

HOMEWORK

- o Identify your Core Values
- o Identify your needs and wants
- o Truly think about how your work and life integrate with each other, then discuss this with a trusted friend.
- o Complete your Wants and Needs Blueprint

REFERENCES

3. Maslow, A. (1943). "A theory of human motivation". Psychological Review. 50 (4): 370-96.

NOTES

Chapter 3

YOUR TEAM OF ADVISORS

Doc: *Why do I NEED a financial advisor, an attorney, an accountant, etc.? I'm smart, so I can figure it out.*

Dr. Bonnie: *Yes, as docs, we are indeed smart. However, we have to make the best use of our limited time, capacity and energy while practicing.*

Just as doctors specialize, professionals in other industries specialize, as well. My recommendation is to leverage the expertise of trusted advisors, after proper vetting, to assist you in making the most informed decisions possible given the limited amount of time that most physicians have to address critical, non-clinical issues in our lives.

In this chapter, our goal is to understand:

o The importance and the process of building your Team of trusted advisors.
o An overview of the role of each Trusted Advisors in working with you and with your entire Team of Trusted Advisors
o That our Trusted Advisors should be education-oriented, because this resonates with our core value of being lifelong learners, aka career nerds.8 Eat Healthily, Exercise and Sleep Well

Building and activating our team of Trusted advisors ultimately helps us to achieve our long-term goals effectively and efficiently. They assist us in navigating the confusing and changing waters in business, financial, legal, and accounting fields.

By smarter, I am referring to:

o Admitting that we don't know what we don't know (I know this is hard for most of us.)
o Using our resources to gain knowledge, including surrounding ourselves with people who know more about a subject than we do
o Building and activating our network's access to gain knowledge from their experiences, empowering us to make critical and informed decisions

As doctors, we engage multi-specialty healthcare teams to address many patient complexities, which acknowledge the inherent strength and effectiveness of integrating the multiplicity of knowledge from several sources. Similarly, when it comes to making decisions concerning the non-clinical, yet critical aspects of being a doctor, we can also build a team of trusted advisors to help us navigate these unfamiliar waters.

Our Team of Trusted Advisors!

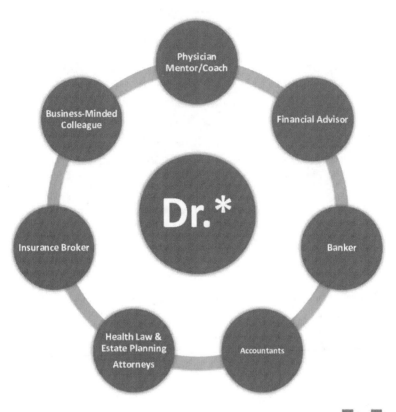

Figure 4 - Power Moves Team of Trusted Advisors

I created this graphic to describe the Circle of Trusted Advisors that we need to assist us in reaching our professional and personal goals, while simultaneously avoiding legal, financial, and tax landmines.

Here we are in the center of this circle, along with our accountability partner, represented by the asterisk. I strongly suggest having a trusted accountability partner, who may be a partner, spouse, friend, or family member, to walk with us as we build our team of advisors.

The accountability partner serves 3 purposes:

- o To support us through this process so that we don't have to build our team alone
- o To help to keep accountable to ensure that we are reaching the goals that we said that we want to reach in the time frame that we want to reach them
- o To serve as an additional set of ears, who are listening and learning from each professional that we interview for positions on our team of advisors

The ultimate goal is to select an advisor from each of these circles who will work with us and each other to make sure that we are encircled with the accurate information that we need to make the best, most-informed decisions possible.

> Red Flag: If an advisor is unwilling to confer and strategize with other members of your Team of Trusted Advisors, then this may be a bad sign.

Trusted advisors are generally willing to share information with other advisors because they too understand that they are not experts in everything. When your advisors confer with one another, this also serves as a checks and balances system for you, which helps us to know that each advisor is doing their part to help us reach our goals. Trusted advisors are knowledgeable and secure in their expertise and should be willing to interface with your other advisors when needed. Advisors who are not willing to confer may have something to hide, so let's keep our eyes and ears open.

For example, when negotiating a contract, doing our due diligence in reviewing the contract requires that we have our trusted advisors review the contract through their specific lens of expertise. During this process, we want our attorney to review the contract, as well as our financial advisor and our accountant. If your financial advisor has a question about the tax implications of one of the signing bonuses being offered, we want the financial advisor to confer with our tax accountant so that together they can recommend how we should negotiate to minimize our tax liability.

When we do not build and engage our Team of Trusted Advisors, we are failing to utilize our most precious commodity of time and energy effectively. We are electing to defer managing the outcomes of having made major business and financial decisions, introducing more chaos into our already hectic, stress-filled lives.

> *Power Move #8* - *All professionals need a coach. We are the star player on our own team, so let's build our team of expert advisors to help us navigate to the finish line, end zone, or 18th hole, effectively and efficiently.*

Indeed, it is our job to suspend the idea that we know everything. We are smart. Yes, we are very smart, and we are experts in our clinical fields of medicine, and in maybe an additional area or two. However, we must admit that we are not experts in every subject.

Let's start building!

Your goals in building a team of Trusted Advisors include:

- o Building professional relationships, ideally long-term ones
- o Creating accountability and shared liability
- o Leveraging expertise to achieve our strategic goals
- o Creating efficiencies to protect our time

When to start building our Team of Trusted Advisors

When teaching on this subject, this is one of the most common questions that I am asked.

Doc: When should I start building my team of advisors?

Dr. Bonnie: Start the process of building your team 18-24 months before your training ends.

First, I want us to understand that building our Team of Trusted Advisors is a process that takes time. Hence, the recommendation to start a year or two before you transition into the workforce. Even then, your team may not be complete, but at least you would have taken the steps in acquiring at least 1-2 of your team members, so all you must do is remain diligent in completing your team.

As an aside, I can confess that I did not address having an estate plan until I was married and had children, but PLEASE do not follow in my footsteps!

Building your Team of Trusted Advisors will require that you and your accountability partner do your own due diligence in researching, interviewing, and vetting 2-3 candidates to serve on your team, which will require a significant amount of time and effort. This is why I suggest that we start building our Team of Trusted Advisors while in training, such that once our salaries increase to six figures, that we are already working with experts we trust and who have provided us with sound, strategic advice even with our five-digit salaries.

Who are the Members of Our Team of Trusted Advisors?

Because the process of building our Team of Trusted Advisors may take years, I'd like to suggest that we start building our team in the following order:

1. Accountability partner to keep us from feeling isolated during this process

2. Physician mentors and coach to ask specific questions based on their experiences
3. Financial Advisor to help us start implementing healthy financial practices
4. Attorney – Health Law attorney to review your contract
5. Tax Accountant to help us strategize and manage six-figure tax liabilities
6. Insurance Broker – to provide insurance protections
7. Banker (Private Wealth Manager) to assist us with our banking needs efficiently
8. Practice Administrator or a Friend/Colleague in Business to run inevitable business or practice decisions by as someone who can give us an alternative viewpoint

So as an overview, let's look at the key questions that we need to ask when we are working to identify the members of our Team of Trusted Advisors using the 5 Ws:

o Who is this advisor & what is their purpose?
o What credentials should these advisors have? What are their core values?
o When do I need to engage this advisor, and in what types of decisions specifically?
o Where can I find or identify candidates for this role on my team?
o Why is this advisor a critical member of the Circle of Trusted Advisors?
o How is this advisor compensated? How does this advisor help me with my contract/negotiations?

Please note that the answers to these key questions are geared towards how the members of your Team of Trusted advisors can support and guide you through contract negotiations. A comprehensive review of each of the advisor's roles, responsibilities, and critical questions to ask will be provided in my pending eBook, *The Doctor's Ultimate Guide to Building Our Team of Trusted Advisors.*

TABLE 1 - ACCOUNTABILITY PARTNER (AP)

Who is this advisor & what is their purpose?	This is a trusted friend, partner, spouse or family member whose opinion you respect and will help to keep you accountable. This person should be responsible and task driven as you are partnering with them to help you reach your goals. This person should also be willing to challenge you if you are not completing your stated tasks.
What credentials should these advisors have? What are their core values?	Your AP may not have specific credentials, but this person should certainly have your respect and possible skills that complement or supplement your areas in need of improvement.
When do I need to engage this advisor, and for what types of decisions specifically?	First and early. Start building your Team of Trusted Advisors by engaging your accountability partner who can help you interview candidates and weigh in on their fit for your team.
Where can I find or identify candidates for this role on my team?	This is a trusted friend, partner, spouse or family member.
Why is this advisor a critical member of the Circle of Trusted Advisors?	Building your Team of Trusted Advisors is a time consuming and arduous task. Your AP is meant to provide you with support, help offset the feelings of isolation, and should be willing to help with scheduling meetings and attend candidate interviews with you.
How is this advisor compensated? How do I know if they are of benefit to me or not?	Your AP is not a paid member of your Circle of Trusted Advisors. You are the only person that can determine whether your AP is being supportive and keeping you accountable.
Other Important Considerations	Experience in the field.

TABLE 2 - PHYSICIAN MENTOR/COACH

Who is this advisor & what is their purpose?	This is a trusted doctor colleague, mentor or sponsor who is willing to transparently share their experiences, best practices and advice with you. If you do not have an organic relationship with such a colleague, you can hire a doctor coach for support.
What credentials should these advisors have? What are their core values?	Your doctor mentors and coaches should reflect your core values and have likely taken a professional pathway as one that you would like to model.
When do I need to engage this advisor, and for what types of decisions specifically?	This advisor should be engaged early and frequently. This advisor should be as objective as possible, although this should be someone that you trust and whose opinions you respect.
Where can I find or identify candidates for this role on my team?	Your AP may not have specific credentials, but this person should certainly have your respect and possible skills that complement or supplement your areas in need of improvement.
Why is this advisor a critical member of the Circle of Trusted Advisors?	Physician mentors and coaches can be identified while in training, in your professional associations or in online affinity groups. Your goal is to build a relationship with this person over time, so that you can engage them when it is time to start making critical decisions.
How is this advisor compensated? How do I know if they are of benefit to me or not?	Physician mentors and coaches have walked in your shoes and can thereby lend advice through the lens of a colleague. The remaining members of your Trusted Advisors may or may not be doctors.
How is this advisor compensated? How do I know if they are of benefit to me or not?	Physician mentors are not compensated members of your team, so we should be respectful of their time and express appreciation. Physician coaches are compensated via hourly rates or flat fees.
Other Important Considerations	You should ideally have more than one doctor mentor.

TABLE 3 - FINANCIAL ADVISOR (FA)

Who is this advisor & what is their purpose?	This Trusted Advisor is a credentialed expert in assisting us, their doctor-clients, in one or more of the following:Building a financial strategyImplementing the financial strategyPurchasing insurance protectionsInvesting It is your job to inquire about each FA's role.
What credentials should these advisors have? What are their core values?	There are over 50 designations that FA's can hold. Some planners may have multiple designations, while others may not have any. • Personal Financial Specialist (PFS) – CPAs can undergo additional financial planning education and after passing meeting exam and experience requirements can use the CPA/PFS designation. • Certified Financial Planner (CFP®) – The CFP is one of the most respected financial planning designations as it requires a minimum of three years of experience, follows a strict code of ethics, and passes a series of three exams. These individuals will be able to provide a broad range of financial advice. • Chartered Financial Consultant (ChFC) – These are typically insurance professionals who specialize in some aspects of financial planning by meeting additional education requirements in economics and investments. • Chartered Retirement Planning Counselor (CRPC) – A CRPC designation is offered through the College of Financial Planning to allow planners to specialize in retirement planning. These individuals must also pass an exam and meet a strict code of ethics.
When do I need to engage this advisor, and for what types of decisions specifically?	This Trusted Advisor should be communicated with frequently and often, ideally before and while you are contemplating any major life changes or transitions. Your FA should review your contract with the goal of helping you calculate the total compensation value of your contract, which includes more than just the salary being offered.
Where can I find or identify candidates for this role on my team?	www.NAPFA.org www.fpanet.org
Why is this advisor a critical member of the Circle of Trusted Advisors?	This is the advisor that should be able to provide financial insight into each decision that we need to make when we are building our financial strategy, transitioning between practices or facing financial challenges.
How do I know if they are of benefit to me or not?	FA's are compensated in one of three ways:flat feescommission from products, i.e. insurance products or assets that clients purchasefees received as a percentage of the total amount of funds or investments that the FA is managing on our behalf.
Other Important Considerations	If you are married, it is important that you and your spouse agree upon, trust, and communicate with your FA. Therefore, it is most helpful to interview this candidate with your spouse too, which will enable you to either begin building a relationship with this person early on, or allow you to veto this candidate if you and your spouse do not agree on this candidate.

TABLE 4 - BANKER (AKA PRIVATE WEALTH MANAGER)

Who is this advisor & what is their purpose?	Physicians are considered to be high net worth individuals secondary to the six-figure incomes that we generate. Most banking institutions have a customer service branch to support high net worth individuals. Depending on the bank, these bankers may be called private wealth managers. These individuals are in place to help facilitate banking activities for their clients alleviating the time required to travel to the bank to carry out routine banking activities.
What credentials should these advisors have? What are their core values?	These bankers should be credentialed through their specific banking institutions. Many have degrees in finance or business. Some may hold similar credentials to FA's.
When do I need to engage this advisor, and for what types of decisions specifically?	This advisor should be able to provide information and options on securing mortgages, home or retail loans. This person may also provide additional savings or investment options offered by their banking institution.
Where can I find or identify candidates for this role on my team?	Your local bank or wealth management firm should be able to direct you to the private wealth management bankers within their bank.
Why is this advisor a critical member of the Circle of Trusted Advisors?	This advisor is critical when it comes to helping you process banking activities with the convenience of being able to take care of most transactions online or via phone.
How is this advisor compensated? How do I know if they are of benefit to me or not?	The bank through which they are employed compensates some bankers. Private wealth managers may be compensated via the same vehicles that FA's are compensated, i.e., flat fees, commission on products sold or commission on assets under management.
Other Important Considerations	Keep your banker/private wealth manager on speed dial!

TABLE 5 - ACCOUNTANT

Who is this advisor & what is their purpose?	Your accountant plays a critical role in communicating your financial practices into the required tax-return and reporting required by the IRS. As your income increases as a doctor in practice, you will want to consult this person(s) frequently and often, ie. to review your contract, before you file your withholding paperwork in a new position, and prior to filing your taxes.
What credentials should these advisors have? What are their core values?	• Certified Public Accountant (CPA) - A CPA is an experienced accountant that has met strict education and licensing requirements. A CPA will be a good choice for tax planning and preparation. • For doctors in private practice or in business, a bookkeeper, who is also a type of accountant will track record and reconcile the business' financial activities on a daily, weekly, monthly, quarterly and annual basis. Your bookkeeper will provide your financials to your tax accountant in order to prepare your annual tax returns. • Enrolled Agents are tax professionals who have passed a rigorous test and background check administered by the IRS. Enrolled agents often specialize and are best for complex tax situations. • A Tax Preparer may be registered by the state. Best for straightforward tax returns. • the national Tax Franchises are H&R Block, Jackson Hewitt, and Liberty Tax. Offices nationwide are often fast, courteous, and convenient.
When do I need to engage this advisor and what type of decisions, specifically?	Engage your accountant when a change in income is anticipated, during major life transitions (marriage, children, divorce), starting a business endeavor, for tax preperation, etc.

Where can I find or identify candidates for this role on my team?	Contact your state's board of accountancy to check the status of a CPA's license, or to find out if any disciplinary action has been taken against the CPA.
	• Personal Referrals
	• American Institute of Certified Public Accountants (AICPA) Directory
	• Business Referrals
	• Accountant Referral Services
	   ○ The Alliance of Cambridge Advisors
	   ○ Garrett Planning Network
	   ○ MyFinancialAdvice.com
	   ○ WiserAdvisor.com
	   ○ Paladin Investor Resources

TABLE 5 - ACCOUNTANT (CONT.)

Why is this advisor a critical member of the Circle of Trusted Advisors?	Your accountant is the key person to help you create a strategic tax plan. Your accountant should also review your contract to help you determine the tax implications of your salary, retirement plan or bonus offers. Your accountant also works on your behalf to keep you out of trouble with the IRS.
How is this advisor compensated? How do I know if they are of benefit to me or not?	Tax accountants may charge a flat fee to prepare your tax return. Bookkeepers likely charge an hourly rate for their bookkeeping services.
Other Important Considerations	Having a bookkeeper and tax accountant who work independently from one another will create a checks and balances system for you, which is an ideal situation. One advisor can weigh in and serve to make sure that the other's practices are professional and accurate.

TABLE 6 - ATTORNEYS (HEALTH, LAW, ESTATE PLANNING, INTELLECTUAL PROPERTY)

Who is this advisor & what is their purpose?	Attorneys specialize just as doctors specialize. Health Law Attorneys specialize in supporting doctors who are transitioning into practice, purchasing a practice, transitioning out of a practice.
What credentials should these advisors have? What are their core values?	These experts will hold a Juris Doctorate (JD) degree and must be licensed to practice law in their respective state by the Bar Association, but certain types of law do not need a bar in that State.) Health lawyers need to know federal and state laws and professional codes, and they should have a healthcare degree or be certified in health care law. The health lawyer that we retain should be an EMPLOYEE-FACING attorney, meaning that this attorney primarily represents physician employees versus employers in their current practice. This is a key question when interviewing health lawyers to potentially serve on your team of advisors.
When do I need to engage this advisor and what type of decisions, specifically?	This is the advisor that will help you discern the legalities of the contract that you are reviewing. This person will work with you to ensure that your needs and ideally your wants are represented in the language of the contract. Your health law attorney can negotiate for you, but only as a backup to you doing your own negotiations.

Where can I find or identify candidates for this role on my team?	The Association of Health Lawyers provides information on health law attorneys. Referrals from colleagues are also a good resource to find helpful legal advisors.
	• American Bar Association (ABA) Lawyer Directory
	• Business Referrals
	• Lawyer Referral Services
	    ○ Nolo's Lawyer Directory
	    ○ The Complete Personal Legal Guide: The Essential Reference for Every Household
	    ○ Consumer's Guide to Legal Help on the Internet

Why is this advisor a critical member of the Circle of Trusted Advisors?	This advisor should take time to understand your goals, objectives, needs, wants, and deal breakers. We partner with our attorneys to ensure that all of the above are included in our contract.
How is this advisor compensated? How do I know if they are of benefit to me or not?	Typical fee arrangements are hourly fees, flat fees, or contingent fees.
Other Important Considerations	Physicians must also engage an estate planning attorney to protect our income and to legally designate and ensure that our wishes are carried out in the case of disability or death. Estate planning attorneys charge a flat fee to implement the 6-7 components of an estate plan, which must be filed in your state of residence.

For Educational Purposes Only. Not Intended as Legal Advice.

TABLE 7 - INSURANCE BROKER

Who is this advisor & what is their purpose?	Although some financial advisors sell insurance, insurance brokers also sell multiple types of insurance that doctors will need to protect our income and property. The types of insurance protections that one might consider include, but are not limited to: • Life-Disability • Homeowners'/Renters' • Property and Casualty • Umbrella Insurance
What credentials should these advisors have? What are their core values?	Your insurance broker will be licensed to sell insurance by the state. This person also has to have passed several certification examinations in order to be licensed to sell insurance, such as a series 7. An insurance broker's credentials and licenses can be verified at www.finra.org.
When do I need to engage this advisor and what type of decisions, specifically?	Work with your FA to determine which insurance protections are warranted for your specific financial situation and strategy
Where can I find or identify candidates for this role on my team?	Commercial insurance agents who work for specific companies are often times limited to selling insurance products their company sells. Insurance brokers usually have the option to offer insurance products from various companies in order to help meet your specific needs. Independent agents are like brokers in that they have the capacity and connections to access insurance policy products that best fit your needs and strategy.
Why is this advisor a critical member of the Circle of Trusted Advisors?	Purchasing protection of our assets is certainly an option that is open to everyone. It is our job to become knowledgeable about the numerous insurance options. Your insurance broker should be interested in educating you on these options prior to presenting you with an opportunity to purchase any policy.
How is this advisor compensated? How do I know if they are of benefit to me or not?	Insurance agents/brokers are primarily paid on commission on insurance products sold.

TABLE 8 - PRACTICE ADMINISTRATOR OR A FRIEND/COLLEAGUE IN BUSINESS

Who is this advisor & what is their purpose?	This is a person who primarily works on the business side of their respective industry. We need this person in our circle to help us evaluate options and advise us through the lens of someone who has been educated on business practice in the way that doctors have not.
What credentials should these advisors have? What are their core values?	This person could be a practice administrator, an executive, an attorney, or other professional who can weigh in on our decisions from a non-doctor perspective
When do I need to engage this advisor, and for what types of decisions specifically?	Having a person who is willing to weigh in on potential advisors or even on financial strategies and decisions is advised. Again this person is in place to offer an alternate point of view to our own.
.Where can I find or identify candidates for this role on my team?	We likely have friends or classmates who pursued careers in fields outside of medicine. You likely know someone that you can integrate into your network to help serve this purpose. Alternatively, this person would also gain from having a trusted healthcare expert on their team, as well.
Why is this advisor a critical member of the Circle of Trusted Advisors?	Non-doctors think differently. People in business fields also speak the same language, just as those in healthcare speak the same language. It is good to have someone in your corner who was trained or has experience in business or in arenas that are different from our own. This diversity of input creates improved outcomes and problem solving. It also helps to curb the notion that we can only take advice from other doctors, which sometimes leads to the blind leading the blind.
How is this advisor compensated? How do I know if they are of benefit to me or not?	This advisor is not a compensated member of your Team of Trusted advisors. You will know if they are of benefit if they offer input and advice that prompts you to think differently.
Other Important Considerations	

How to Start Building your Team of Trusted Advisors

With regards to each prospective Trusted Advisor, we must do our due diligence, which can be described as taking the following steps:

1. Identify 3-5 candidates
   a. Consider having Trusted Advisors who work for/with different institutions, and those who have or specialize in working with doctors
2. Research candidates online
3. Interview 2-3 candidates
4. Check 2-3 referrals for each candidate
5. Follow up with the candidate who was decided upon during your final selection and set a date for the first meeting
6. Prepare for this meeting by having your documents in order, starting with our <u>Master Organization List for Trainees</u> and a separate <u>Master Organization List for Practicing Physicians</u> (See Appendix D & E).
7. Complete your <u>Power Moves Team of Trusted Advisors Tracker</u> (See Section 1, Power Moves Workbook)

Yes, this is a time-consuming process, so along with your accountability partner, you may want to set the goal of identifying 2-3 candidates over an 8-week period. Such a timeline would enable you to build your entire team in 18-24 months.

STEP 1 - IDENTIFYING CANDIDATES FOR YOUR CIRCLE OF TRUSTED ADVISORS

Consult with the following entities to begin identifying 3-5 candidates for each member of your Trusted Advisors Team:

o   Physician colleagues and online forums
o   Local or State Medical Societies
o   Associations for specific industries, e.g., the Health Lawyers Association

STEP 2 - RESEARCHING CANDIDATES

Reviewing the candidate's online profile on their website, the website of their professional association, and their LinkedIn, Facebook, and/or Twitter is extremely important. While you cannot trust everything that you read online, you should take time to become familiar with this individual and their character prior to having your first meeting with them. Be sure to look for referrals and reviews from other healthcare professionals, as well.

STEP 3 - INTERVIEWING PROSPECTIVE CANDIDATES

Keep in mind that your #1 goal is to start building a professional relationship with an advisor that you can come to trust. Relationship building takes time and may require more than a conversation with the candidate initially, as you work to determine whether this person could be a good fit for you and your team.

Your first interview with a potential advisor should serve as a "Discovery" session. If possible, attend this initial meeting in person and with your accountability partner. During this first call or meeting, you want to learn as much about this person as possible in this short period of time, and vice versa.

You are listening for expertise, experience, emphasis on education, patience, tolerance, willingness to teach, alignment with your core values. Be sure to ask:

- o for examples of how the candidate works best with clients to achieve their goals
- o about what is expected from you as the client
- o what you can expect from them
- o about the benefits that clients have received
- o about the best modes of communication
- o potential downsides or negative outcomes

> Red Flag: Any attempt to make sales or solicit purchases during an initial discovery session is a Red Flag.

STEP 4 - CHECKING REFERENCES

If you are reasonably satisfied with the interaction with the candidate, following this initial meeting, we need to check the references that the candidate provided. This is a security step that provides some level of protection and should NOT be skipped. Checking references can save us time, money, and emotional distress in the long run.

Exception: Lawyers cannot give references as it would be a breach in attorney-client privilege.

> **Power Move #9** - Just as we do not base our research conclusions based on data collected from a sample size with an n =1, we have to check multiple references for each advisor, including those from other professionals and from other doctor-clients.

Not checking references can be extremely detrimental. I have had many docs call to share their disappointment or disgust about their advisors with me. Yet, when I inquired about whether the doc had checked the advisor's references, of course, the doc had not checked them.

Simply put, we cannot be angry about things we do not ask about. We must do our due diligence.

Figure 5 is a sample of an email communication that I use when checking references for trusted advisors, consultants, or employees.

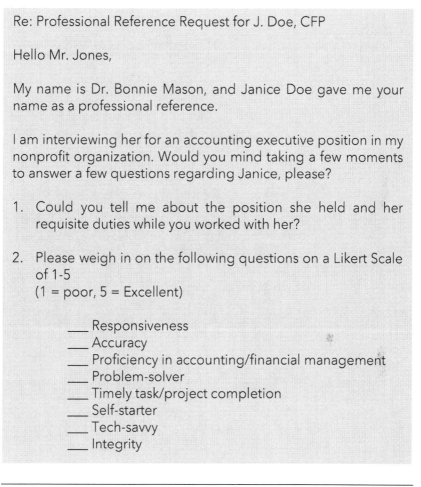

Re: Professional Reference Request for J. Doe, CFP

Hello Mr. Jones,

My name is Dr. Bonnie Mason, and Janice Doe gave me your name as a professional reference.

I am interviewing her for an accounting executive position in my nonprofit organization. Would you mind taking a few moments to answer a few questions regarding Janice, please?

1. Could you tell me about the position she held and her requisite duties while you worked with her?

2. Please weigh in on the following questions on a Likert Scale of 1-5
    (1 = poor, 5 = Excellent)

    ___ Responsiveness
    ___ Accuracy
    ___ Proficiency in accounting/financial management
    ___ Problem-solver
    ___ Timely task/project completion
    ___ Self-starter
    ___ Tech-savvy
    ___ Integrity

Figure 5 - Sample Email for Advisor or Vendor Reference Checks

Most professionals who serve as references will likely respond to your email inquiry within 24-48 hours.

Part of doing your due diligence is remaining alert and aware of potential Red Flags and warning signs, many of which may center around communication. If your Spidey-sense is tingling, then you may want to pay closer attention and ask more questions.

STEPS 5 & 6 - SELECTING MEMBERS OF YOUR TEAM OF TRUSTED ADVISORS

Now that we have completed our due diligence, it is time to select our Trusted Advisor team members by following up with each candidate to let them know whether we have elected to work with them or not. Don't forget to set the date, time, and location for your first meeting with the advisor with the agenda and items that you need to provide.

> Red Flag: Selecting family members and/or close friends to serve as your Trusted Advisors introduces specific challenges to this already arduous process. Just note that our personal relationships can be damaged if something goes wrong. It is important to make an honest assessment as to whether comprising your relationship with this person is worth it.

STEP 7 - DOCUMENT AND SHARE

Then, completing your Trusted Advisors Tracker, which contains the contact info of your Team of Trusted Advisors is mandatory, and should be shared with your accountability partner in case of an emergency. See for your Trusted Advisors Tracker.(Section 1, Power Moves Workbook)

When to Engage your Team of Trusted Advisors

By taking the following actions after selecting members of your team of advisors, you will maximize the efficiency in making some of life's tough decisions.

> **Power Move #10** - *Meet with your Trusted Advisors frequently, e.g. quarterly to semi-annually. Once you articulate your desire to meet routinely, your Trusted Advisor should be proactively working to engage you per your desire.*

> **Power Move #11** - *Consult your Trusted Advisors when making ALL career, leadership, business, practice management, legal, and financial decisions.*

> **Power Move #12** - *When reviewing contracts, allow time for each of your trusted advisors to review the agreement from their perspective, which gives you a comprehensive analysis of the potential opportunity.*

At the end of the day, we have a choice as to how we will contend with making the career, leadership, business, practice management, and the plethora of financial decisions that will affect our current lives and our family's legacy.

CHAPTER SUMMARY

POWER MOVES

- Build your Team of Trusted Advisors, starting with your accountability partner(s)
- Work smarter, not harder by building and routinely engaging with members of your Team of Trusted Advisors.
  - Meet with your Trusted Advisors frequently, quarterly to semi-annually. Once you articulate your desire to meet routinely, your Trusted Advisor should be proactively working to engage you.
- Always check the references provided by prospective Trusted Advisor candidates. Follow the recommended 7-Step Process for Building Your Team
- Your Trusted Advisors should be willing to work with one another on your behalf to ensure that YOUR comprehensive strategies and goals for your professional and personal lives are being met.
- Our Trusted Advisors should be education-oriented, because this resonates with our core value of being lifelong learners, aka career nerds.
- Consider having Trusted Advisors who work for/with different institutions and companies as a checks and balances move, and those who have or specialize in working with doctors for quality assurance
- Consult your Trusted Advisors when making ALL career, leadership, business, practice management, legal, and financial decisions
- When reviewing contracts, allow time for each of your trusted advisors to review the agreement from their perspective, which gives you a comprehensive analysis of the potential opportunity.

RED FLAGS

- Your mother's brother's cousin's sister is most likely not the best candidate to serve as one of your Trusted Advisors.
- When a Trusted Advisor is unwilling to work with your other advisors, there is likely a reason.

o Any advisor that encourages you to make a purchase or investment during your initial encounters with them, beware.
o Slow or untimely responsiveness to your inquiries as the client is troubling.
o Lack of industry-standard credentials or those which cannot be verified publicly is also problematic.

HOMEWORK

o Meet with your accountability partner to begin setting up the timeline for selecting your team of trusted advisors
o Complete your <u>Power Moves Team of Trusted Advisors Tracker</u> in Section 1 of your Power Moves Workbook and share it with your accountability partner, in case of an emergency.
o Set up standing meeting dates with your accountability, at least once per month until you have successfully built your team of advisors

NOTES

_____

_____

_____

_____

_____

_____

_____

_____

_____

_____

_____

_____

Chapter 4

TOP 10 CONTRACT MISTAKES DOCTORS MAKE

Doc: *Quick question - Which contract mistakes should I avoid?*

Dr. Bonnie: *I am SO happy that you asked this question, but there are no quick answers to this question.*

Hopefully, this book will serve as a starting point!

The goal of this chapter is to describe the most common mistakes that doctors make when it comes to contracts and negotiations. This list is based on the thousands of doctors that I have taught and the hundreds of doctors that I have personally mentored and strategized with over the past 15 years.

TOP 10 CONTRACT MISTAKES THAT PHYSICIANS SHOULD AVOID

Mistake #1 - We often do not read our contracts, because we are just hoping that everything will be okay.

The very first mistake is one that is the easiest to correct with a simple shift of our mindset, and I absolutely want to curb the notion that we can just sign the contract while HOPING that everything will be okay.

Hope, alone, is not a contract negotiation strategy!

Certainly, just the thought of sifting through a 25-page document that we have received no education about is completely daunting, but this way of thinking can end, right here and now.

The purpose of this book is to provide enough background and foundational information so that we can become more educated and empowered to read and derive an understanding of this powerful document, despite the feelings of anxiety and discomfort that the thought of reviewing an employment contract elicits.

So, welcome to your discomfort zone of contracts and negotiations!

Discomfort zones are not new to us, let's think of this as starting a new clinical rotation. Even though we may not have been familiar with the specialty, we showed up on the wards ready to learn.

Trust me, we can attack learning about contracts with the same trepid eagerness, and we can be successful.

The cost of not reading our contracts thousands of dollars from potential:

- o lost income
- o early or unexpected transition costs
- o potential legal fees
- o negative impact on our professional careers, credentials or licensing
- o negative impact on our personal lives and family

If for no other reason, after learning to read and negotiate our contracts, we can now have a voice and impact on our own future.

When we are better informed→ we make better decisions → and we live our best lives, which benefits us, our families and certainly our patients.

Mistake #2 – We sign our contracts too quickly!

Usually under pressure and time constraints given by the potential employer or its representative, many doctors wind up signing the contract as presented, sometimes within days of receiving it. This is an absolute no-no, no thank you, and please don't.

Being pressured from an external entity to sign the contract satisfies their needs, but not necessarily ours. We should not sign any contract in haste because an accelerated time frame does not give us enough time to do our due diligence and have the contract reviewed by our "Team of Trusted Advisors."

Signing our contracts too quickly can cost us thousands of dollars because it does not allow us time to:

- o Consider how we can negotiate our individual needs and wants into the contract
- o Compare multiple employment opportunities simultaneously
- o Research and negotiate for fair market compensation in that particular region

    o Do our due diligence by having our trusted advisors review our contract

Realistically and in my experience while coaching hundreds of doctors through this process, reasonable contract negotiations can take anywhere from 2-6 months, from the time you receive the agreement through final negotiations and signatures. So, let's breathe and take our time.

When you encounter an entity that frowns upon you taking the time to do your due diligence, RUN!

> **Power Move #13** - *We are no longer going to make six-figure decisions in five days.*

Mistake #3 – We don't have our contracts reviewed by our trusted advisors.

Not having our contracts reviewed by attorneys and our other advisors is a huge mistake because of the potential professional, legal, and financial consequences to practice lie within an employment contract.

For most of us, an employment contract represents a body of information where "we don't know what we don't know," which makes the prospect of having to read, review, and discuss this document that much more intimidating and daunting.

However, these are the very reasons that we should take the time to assemble our team of trusted advisors who serve as subject-matter experts as well as individually and collectively advise us on the unknown impact that the contract can have on our professional and personal lives.

Not having our contracts reviewed by our trusted advisors can cost us:

- o legally
- o financially when it comes to understanding benefits, taxes and accounting
- o professionally

If you want to go fast, go alone. If you want to go far, go together!
~African Proverb

Mistake #4 – Some of us are obstinate, stubborn or frustrated when it comes to learning about contracts. I often hear doctors say things like, "I didn't go to medical school to learn the business of medicine, and I refuse to spend my time doing so. I'll just have an attorney tell me if this is a good contract."

The thought of reviewing and analyzing a contract can be overwhelming for anyone, and especially for doctors since understanding the business of medicine was not what we anticipated.

As a result, many doctors who have taken the next step to retain an attorney (Yay!) have entrusted the attorney with telling them whether this is a good contract or not. (No!) There's more to it than that.

Yes, an attorney can tell us whether a contract is legally sound. However, unless we have taken the time to assess and share our needs and wants with the attorney, that attorney cannot tell us whether this is a good contract FOR US.

Just as doctors appreciate having patients who are informed and who want to be engaged participants in the doctor-patient relationship. Similarly, we need to be the informed client when we are working with our attorney, financial advisor, accountant, or banker in order to make the best decisions for ourselves, as well. When we know what we need and want, this helps our advisors give us the best, customized advice that will help us reach our personal and financial goals. Then, we can approach our contract negotiations with confidence, because we are now informed and well-advised. This is working smarter, not harder!

In short, the cost of shying away from learning this information is astronomical, and can lead to multiple job transitions, financial instability, stress, disempowerment and disruptions in our professional and personal lives.

> **Power Move #14** - *Let's learn how to analyze our contracts, so that we can confer with our health law attorney, financial advisor and accountant as an informed client, so that we can develop an informed and strategic approach to our contract negotiations.*

Mistake #5 - Most times, we don't ask enough questions, primarily because we don't know what we don't know.

When it comes to contracts, negotiations, finances, and other non-clinical aspects of medicine, we certainly don't always know what questions to ask. However, we have to first take on the mindset that there is no dumb question when it comes to learning about the subjects that we were not taught in medical school or in training. Just think about it, these are not our fields of expertise, but there are important questions that we need to ask when it comes to the contract.

When discussing our contracts with our advisors, one approach to asking questions in these arenas is using an "If...then..." approach, especially when discussing unfamiliar topics or subjects. Because we don't know what we don't know, we don't often understand the consequences or ramifications of what we are agreeing to once we sign the contract.

Here are a couple of examples of ways to formulate "If..., then..." questions around unfamiliar or nebulous topics or contract terms:

1. An employment contract requires that a specific number of relative value units (RVUs) are being required in order to qualify for a productivity bonus. Here are two "If..., then..."question that you could subsequently ask is:

"If I generate the required number of RVUs, then how is the productivity bonus calculated?"

"If I don't generate this specific number of RVUs, then what are the consequences?"

2. You are negotiating for relocation costs with your potential employer as a part of your total compensation package, and you are discussing the financial and tax implications within the contract with your accountant. In this example, an appropriate question to ask might be,

    "If the amount of the relocation costs is paid directly to me vs. directly to the moving company, then what will the tax implications be in either case?"

If we don't ask enough questions, then we can't be surprised when we are reaping the consequences of something that we signed up for unknowingly. It is our job to ask as many questions as we can to manage our expectations as a part of doing our due diligence.

Just to reinforce this point, my former chair and mentor once reinforced this point with me, when encouraging me to ask more questions until I achieved clarity:

"We've been in school for a long time, so there isn't too much that we shouldn't be able to understand once a new concept is being explained. If someone is not willing to educate you in terms that you understand, then they either don't understand it themselves or they are indicating that they may not want to work with you. If either is the case, then don't do business with this person." Sage advice. Let's take heed!

The cost of not asking questions on any number of levels can be devastating.

The only dumb question is the one that goes unasked.

Mistake #6 – We don't do our due diligence.

First of all, what is due diligence?

I compare the concept of doing our due diligence to the process of researching and compiling data when we are conducting a research project.

When it comes to contracts, doing our due diligence requires that we take time to learn about and do in-depth research in areas, such as:

- o taking time to reflect and devise a specific list of our needs and wants
- o identifying at least 2 - 3 potential practices or employment opportunities
- o conferring with and reviewing our contracts with our trusted advisors

Unfortunately, delayed gratification, complexity of contracts, and the enigmatic nature of the negotiations process, many of us would prefer avoiding all of the above.

Ultimately, the reason why we should do our due diligence is so that we can apply a data-driven, informed decision-making process to securing the best position for ourselves, which thereby benefits our families and our patients, as well.

Let's be clear, it is the employer's job to get as much for as little as possible. Reciprocally, it is your job to do your due diligence, know your worth, know average RVUs, generate it for the top 10 procedures that you do, know your RVU conversion rate, know what the average number of patients are being seen in your particular specialty in that type of practice setting.

The cost of not doing our due diligence does not only cost us financially, but it often results in loss of time and progress in achieving our goals leading to anxiety and frustration.

Never, EVER sign the first contract that is offered! (We will talk about why.)

Let's do our due diligence first and be sure to negotiate thereafter!

Mistake #7 – Some of us find ourselves practicing with no contract in place at all.

One of the most concerning contract mistakes that doctors make is to practice without a contract in place at all. The most serious call I received was from a doctor who was working without a contract, and her employer stopped paying her and the other doctors. Without a contract in place, they had no written documentation about the back pay they were owed. It was a devastating situation.

Your contract serves to document the details of the rights, protections, obligations, and commitments that the employer is making to you, and vice versa, those that you are making to the employer. If there is no contract, then there is no documentation of said rights, protections, obligations, and commitments, which means the employer cannot necessarily be held responsible or accountable.

No contract = No protections

In addition, if you need to renegotiate an aspect of your employment, such as your compensation, duties, or on-call responsibilities, without a contract, there is no baseline documentation of the initial terms to be renegotiated.

Also, in light of the numbers of hospital mergers and acquisitions in healthcare, we cannot work without a contract. You must insist on having some documentation in writing, i.e., a letter of engagement or commitment, a term sheet, a scope of work or services agreement. We must have our rights, obligations, and commitments in black and white to protect yourself professionally, both now and for your future career.

Exception: If a physician works with no contract in place, then an agreement could be interpreted as IMPLIED, and implied contracts can be binding. When facing this situation, request a copy of the organization's Employee Handbook, which should outline the employer's obligations, policies and procedures for all employees. Read this handbook to glean an understanding of the employer's obligations and commitments to all of its employees as this may be the only document to refer to for future reference.

The cost of working without a contract or document of any kind cannot be enumerated.

If it's not in black and white, it doesn't count nor matter.

Mistake #8 – We fail to encourage our younger physicians to learn the basic business and financial fundamentals.

Discussing business and finances in medicine has long been deemed to be taboo, unprofessional, non-patient centered, and selfish. Instead, we have been conditioned to look at life primarily through the narrow lens of rendering patient care. #stayfocused.

The downside of this narrow approach is that we subsequently fall prey to many business and financial decisions that are either made for us. Why? Many of us have not been equipped with the information, tools, and resources necessary to apply our well-known informed decision-making process to business and finances.

The good news is because we are career nerds, we absolutely can digest and master business concepts and financial fundamentals. Just as we have learned complex pathophysiological processes and surgical techniques, we most certainly have transferable skills and the capacity to understand the business of medicine.

Let's learn the business and financial sides of medicine, starting now!

Mistake #9 – We tend to concentrate on the salary offer in a contract, first and foremost.

When I survey young doctor audiences on what is the most important aspect of the contract, "the salary" is by far the most common response that I receive.

As will be pointed out repeatedly in this book, while important, the salary offer is NOT the most important term in our employment agreement. In fact, please pay close attention to the list of the top five contract terms, which tend to turn into landmines for doctors in Chapter 8. It is imperative that all doctors understand the top five terms that tend to cause doctors the most distress.

The cost of only concentrating on the salary can result in leaving tens of thousands of dollars that we could have negotiated for, from missed benefits, leave, pay for call and other expenses that perhaps could be covered if we would only ask for what we need and want.

It's NOT all about the Benjamins, Baby!

Mistake #10 – We are unclear about the finality and ramifications of signing our contracts.

Before you sign the contract, this document outlines a list of expectations, options and opportunities, rights and protections that can be negotiated.

Prior to signing the contract is the time at which you have the most leverage, i.e., the greatest ability to negotiate.

However, after the contract is signed by both parties, i.e., executed, this becomes a document comprised of legally enforceable commitments and obligations. Also, keep in mind that renegotiating your contract after it has been signed is often less successful, requires a sound strategy, and may require that you retain additional legal counsel.

Therefore, it is critical that we understand the expectations, options, rights, and protections first. Then, we must negotiate the best terms possible prior to signing the contract.

The goal is to negotiate a final contract which represents the best interests of both the employer and the employee. Therefore, we must negotiate before we sign the contract, for doing so afterwards can cost us thousands of dollars.

CHAPTER SUMMARY

POWER MOVES

- o Let's learn how to analyze our contracts so that we can confer with our health law attorney as an informed client, just as we appreciate partnering with informed patients.
- o We are no longer going to make six-figure decisions in five days.
- o We will ask questions until we achieve clarity and understanding, even when it makes us feel uncomfortable or when we think this is something we SHOULD know. Ask!!!

TAKE-HOME POINTS

- o Please learn from these mistakes that other doctors have made in order to protect yourself, your family, your career, and your patients.

RED FLAGS

- o Respectfully disengage from those who might tell you that you do not have to learn about the business/financial aspects of medicine. These might be the same people who tell you that you don't need a lawyer. This may have been true in the past, but the corporatization of medicine in the last decade is only projected to increase in the next decade. My advice to you...let's learn all that we can in these areas.

HOMEWORK

- o Take a moment to reflect on which of these top contract mistakes you have made or have the potential to make. Use these mistakes to catalyze your willingness to learn about contracts, business, and financial aspects of medicine.

NOTES

_____

_____

_____

_____

_____

_____

_____

_____

_____

_____

_____

_____

_____

_____

_____

_____

_____

_____

_____

_____

_____

Chapter 5

THE ANATOMY OF A CONTRACT

Doc: *I have never read a contract before, and I have no idea where or how to start. I am getting nauseous just thinking about it.*

Dr. Bonnie: *No worries. After all of these years, reading contracts can still raise my anxiety level a bit. Let's compare this to a subject that we are more familiar with, such as anatomy, and keep an open mind, Doc. We can do this!*

Becoming familiar with a contract requires practice, and with repetition, a greater understanding and a decreased sense of anxiety can result. Remember, the more we presented patients on rounds, the easier it became?

Adult learners need three things in order to retain new information:

1. Relevance
2. Rigor
3. Repetition

The goal of this chapter is to gain an understanding of only three core components or parts of a contract as a starting point.

Thus, for the sake of repetition, I am going to compare the components of a contract to parts of the human anatomy to ease the digestion of this material.

Employment Agreements &/or Contracts

Before diving into a anatomical discussion, let's answer a common question, "What is the difference between an employment agreement and an employment contract?"

EMPLOYMENT <u>AGREEMENT</u> - A formal agreement that spells out the rules of engagement between an employee and an employer. Compensation and expectations and benefits are typical subjects. Known generally as employment contracts, they are time-limited, viable for a specified period, e.g. one year.

EMPLOYMENT <u>CONTRACT</u> - An agreement between an employer and an employee. It is typically voluntary, deliberate, and legally enforceable, therefore, binding. The employee must agree to this contract as a condition of his/her employment. Employment contracts cover a variety of procedures and/or policies that are required for the employer to protect its own interest. The contract often states a time frame inhibiting the employee from working for a competitor or in a similar industry after they leave the company. This section is often contested in the courts.

Yes, these definitions are quite similar, and in fact, the terms employment contract and employment agreement are often used interchangeably, as you will see throughout this book.

As an employee, your primary responsibilities to your employer are to carry out the clinical, administrative, and teaching responsibilities that will be outlined in your contract. It is important to understand that your employee contract (agreement) is binding, which means that upon signing by both yourself and the employer, you are agreeing to every term in the document. Now we can delve into the core of this chapter.

Three Anatomical Components of a Contract

We will start building our understanding of a contract by defining three key contractual components of a contract by literally using gross anatomical references.

(At the risk of being too literal in this description of the parts of the contract, I will share a few additional comparisons to the human anatomy as a basis of reference in Appendix F, the Power Moves Anatomy of a Contract, Extended Version. My husband thought the additional references were a bit too much, and they may be. However, in the spirit of turning contracts into fun concepts, please indulge me when you have a moment. Then, let me know what you think of the anatomical references in Appendix F. Were they helpful or nah? ☺ *Please let me know via email at info@beyondtheexamroom.co.)*

The Face of the Contract - A person's face is our first point of interpersonal engagement. One's face helps us distinguish one person from another, and it allows us to identify a person in the future because of specific facial features.

Similarly, the first section/paragraph in any contract literally serves to define and identify the people, places, and entities that are engaging in a specific contractual arrangement. It contains the key definitions and references relevant to the entire contract.

This first paragraph should not be glossed over or ignored because it contains the following distinctive definitions, which will be referenced throughout the entirety of the remainder of the contract:

- The type of contract or agreement being presented
- The parties who are entering the agreement, such as:
  - the Employer and Physician
  - the Hospital and the Contractor
  - the Lessee and Lessor
- The names, addresses, and corporate structure of the entities
  - Be sure to identify the addresses and/or locations of the
    medical center, which would also be defined in this initial paragraph, as many employers have multiple office locations or satellites that may unknowingly apply to you.
- Dates relevant to the agreement

Here is a sample of the language found in the first paragraph of a fictional employment agreement:

> This PHYSICIAN EMPLOYMENT AGREEMENT is entered into by and between ABC Medical Center, a Maryland professional corporation with multiple locations in multiple states (hereinafter referred to as "Practice"),and Janice Doe, MD (hereinafter referred to as "Physician"), on the following terms and conditions.

In this example, the contract type is being identified, along with the two entities that are engaging in the agreement. This sounds simple enough, but it can become confusing later in the contract if references are made to multiple locations or multiple parties, such as the ABC Medical Center, which has multiple locations in multiple states. This is a critical set of details for us to understand, especially when it comes to a contract's Covenant Not to Compete clause, which will be discussed at length in Chapter 8.

Regardless of the type of contract or agreement, the first paragraph always outlines who the parties are in the proposed arrangement. So please take a moment to circle, underline, and highlight the who, where, and what that will be referred to throughout the contract for yourself first.

The Body of the Contract – Just as the human body houses all major organ systems, the body of a contract houses the main "terms" or "clauses" that govern the two parties entering into the agreement. Based on my experience having read hundreds of physician employment contracts, there are standard "terms" that are generally found in every contract.

Though sometimes the names of these contract terms vary, standard contracts should include and address the following important terms listed here:

Contract Terminology

The most important contract terms for doctors to understand are listed below.

- o Definitions
- o Employment
- o Term and Termination*
- o Duties and Responsibilities*
- o Professional Liability (Malpractice) Insurance*
- o Covenant Not to Compete*
- o Non-Disclosure/Non-Solicitation
- o Intellectual Property/ Outside Revenue*
- o Effect of Termination
- o Ownership Opportunity
- o Compensation
  - o Salary
  - o Leave – Education, Vacation, Sick, Personal time
  - o Fringe Benefits*

      o Moving Costs
      o Loan Repayment, Loan Forgiveness

Additional Terms to be reviewed with your health law attorney

      o Assignability
      o Indemnification
      o Reasonableness of Restrictions
      o Action by Authority with Legal Jurisdiction
      o Representations of Physician
      o Insurance
      o Books, Records, and Office Equipment
      o Notices
      o Severability
      o Waiver
      o Governing Law; Jurisdiction; Venue
o SIGNATURES

In Chapter 8, we will discuss the meanings of these terms, including the Top Contract Terms* that all doctors should know, which are indicated with an asterisk above.

Taking the anatomical analogies a bit further, by equating the "Top 5 Contract Terms that Every Doctor Should Know" to 5 major organ systems. Interpreted very loosely:

    o   Term and Termination → Cardiothoracic System
    o   Non-Compete Clause → Nervous System
    o   Malpractice Insurance → Gastrointestinal System
    o   Fringe Benefits → Integument
    o   Intellectual Property/Outside Revenue Generation → Genitourinary System

Based on my experience, these are the contract terms that cause doctors the most stress and anxiety while transitioning into or between practices. These unforeseen landmines can wreak havoc in the lives of physicians, no matter how much we are being compensated. This is the very reason why compensation is being discussed following the "TOP 5" so that we can build a more comprehensive understanding of our contract that is not limited to a focus on compensation.

Yet, the importance of understanding the compensation model that is being used to calculate our compensation is also critical. Therefore, compensation and physician compensation models topics will be discussed extensively in their own standalone chapter, Chapter 9.

The Extremities of a Contract - This leads us to the final section on compensation, which has purposefully been placed at the end of the contracts terminology discussion. This deprioritization of compensation is intentional, so that we can focus our understanding on the aforementioned terms, and of course, we will pay ample attention to the compensation package being offered. We just don't want to do that first!

Anatomically, our extremities power our musculoskeletal system, literally propelling our bodies and enabling us to move as we choose.

Similarly, I suggest that we can view the compensation components of the contract as the terms provide the fuel we need to power our professional and personal activities.

In some contracts, especially those from academic and large health system employers, the compensation model being offered may be found in the appendix or in the exhibits at the very end of the contract.

Commonly, the appendix or exhibit may contain details pertaining to the:

- o Details regarding compensation and the compensation model that you will be performing under (see Chapter 9 for detailed descriptions of compensation models)
- o Base and possibly variable pay
- o Benefits package

Additionally, the appendix will serve as the location of additional, customized documents for the prospective employee, that serve as supplements or addendums to the primary contract, such as:

- o Promissory note – a loan agreement that specifies the loan, interest, and repayment details of any loans offered as part of the doctor's compensation package.
    - o Signing bonuses, relocation payments or reimbursements, and loan repayment packages are more commonly being offered by employers as repayable loans with interest based on the term (length) of the physician's employment.
    - o Therefore, you must clearly understand the repayment ramifications if you accept one or all of these loans, and you subsequently have to terminate your contract before the entire loan has been repaid. You will likely be required to repay the balance of the loan with interest in one lump sum as a result of terminating the contract.
    - o PLEASE review every page of the contract, including the promissory note with your tax accountant and your financial advisor to determine your tax liability and whether accepting these loans works to your advantage financially.
- o Income guarantee - This type of compensation model is frequently used when rural or underserved communities are looking to recruit physicians into their community to set up a practice. Be extremely careful when considering practicing under this model, as the name income guarantee can be a misnomer. I found that many physicians who agree to this model do not understand the complexities nor the associated financial liabilities. ALWAYS review this model in detail with your health law attorney and your personal accountant.
- o Carve Out List for Intellectual Property (See Appendix I) – This addendum serves to notify the employer that the items on this list represent the body of your past, current, and future creative works that you own as your intellectual

property. This list is necessary in order to protect your property and current or future revenues derived from your IP.

Finally, another component of a contract, which is NOT a standard part of every contract is a side letter. A side letter is a separate letter, which may be added to the end of a contract, usually drafted to include the negotiated and agreed upon terms of the contract that are not represented in the body of the contract.

o   Many of the physicians that I have coached have been told, "We don't negotiate the terms of our standard employment contract."
o   This is fine because you can respond by saying, "I completely understand; however, I would like to discuss placing the following negotiated terms in a side letter to accompany the full contract."
o   The side letter should be drafted by YOUR health law attorney so that it will include the agreed-upon negotiated terms as a supplement to the formal contract.
o   Note: Organizations do NOT have to agree to the inclusion of a side letter as a part of your negotiations, but we can present it as a tool for documenting negotiated items, in lieu of changing or editing parts of the master contract.

> *Power Move #15 - Before you begin reading any contract, review the entire document to assess the different components of the contract, i.e., the face, the body, and the appendices/addendums.*

Now, we can move on to analyzing the contract since we now have an understanding of these three parts of the contract in mind:

o   The face, which specifies the who, what, and where of the parties described throughout the agreement
o   The body, which contains the main terms of the contract

o   The extremities, which describe the compensation model and the compensation package

> ***Power Move #16*** *- Verify that all pages included are in sequential order and that no pages are missing from the document, both before and after you sign.*

Hopefully, using this anatomical approach to understanding the primary components of contracts helps! We will be taking a deeper dive into the meaning of these contract terms in Chapter 8, but first, I want to suggest a strategic approach as to how we can analyze and digest our contracts to prevent us from feeling so overwhelmed.

CHAPTER SUMMARY

POWER MOVES

o   Before you begin reading any contract, review the entire document to assess the different components of the contract, i.e., the face, the body, and the appendices/addendums.
o   Verify that all pages included are in sequential order and that no pages are missing from the document, both before and after you sign.

RED FLAGS

o   Always, always, always read the appendices/addendums to the contract. Many vital details hide here.
o   At the end of the contract process, in addition to obtaining signatures from both parties, insist on having both parties initial each page, along with any manual corrections that need to be made.

HOMEWORK

o   Time to practice – Refer to the sample contract that I have provided in Section 2 of your Power Moves Personal Workbook, in order to identify the face, body, and appendages of a contract. This should be a 5-minute or less exercise.

NOTES

_____

_____

_____

_____

_____

_____

_____

_____

_____

_____

_____

_____

_____

_____

_____

_____

_____

_____

_____

_____

_____

_____

For Educational Purposes Only. Not Intended as Legal Advice.

Chapter 6

HOW TO READ YOUR CONTRACT BY TAKING A RISC™

Doc: *Hi Dr. Bonnie, I just signed my contract!*

Dr. Bonnie: *Awesome. Did you review it yourself?*

Doc: *No, I just had a friend who is a real estate attorney review it. They said it was fine.*

Dr. Bonnie: *Silence.* 🙁

The goal of this chapter is to describe a process for analyzing a contract to make understanding contract terms less cumbersome and more digestible.

> **Power Move #17** - *In order to build this new and critically important skill set, I recommend that every doctor read or earnestly attempt to read their own contract first, in preparation for discussing the contract with our health law attorney and our other trusted advisors.*

This chapter is also one of the most empowering chapters in this book, in my humble opinion, because it discusses a contract analysis strategy that has been successfully utilized by so many doctors that I have coached over the years. Given this fact, I am confident that each of us can become more comfortable with analyzing and reviewing our own contracts utilizing this plan and with practice.

Before the Analyzing Begins

Even now, after having reviewed hundreds and hundreds of contracts over the past 2 decades, the thought of sitting down to review any contract requires that I coach myself and settle my nerves by reassuring myself that, "I can do this!" and you can, too. Here's how:

1. First, let's breathe.
2. Prepare your physical space. Please prepare to review your contract by taking out your highlighter or by tapping your highlighter function so that we can prepare to annotate and highlight key areas within each term of the contract. I liken analyzing contracts to studying for board exams or other standardized exams. I sit in a well-lit environment with minimal distractions. I have my highlighters and colored tabs ready with a hard copy of the contract in front of me, and now I'm all set.

3. I double check to make sure that I have my Need and Wants Blueprint available as a quick reference during my analysis.
4. Let's take another breath. Here we go!

Power Move #18 - *Analyzing a contract comes after reflecting on your needs and wants from Chapter 2.*

The Big Picture – Take a RISC using the RISC Analysis™

When it comes to understanding your contract, we will first delve into HOW to analyze your contract and its common terms using a contracts analysis framework that I developed about 7 years ago called the RISC Analysis™.

Because I was at the point where I was reading 1-2 contracts a month as a physician coach, which later increased to 1-2 contracts per week, I needed an approach or formula that would help to decrease my own anxiety when it comes to contracts. In developing my approach, I also needed to answer the following questions:

o How could I attack each term in the contract?
o What infrastructure, outline, or approach could I use to analyze each term within the contract to decrease the anxiety that I feel while attempting to read a document with no previous training or education on how to do so?

Subsequently, the RISC Analysis™ was born.

This wasn't a complete surprise because as a chemistry major with a mathematics minor at Howard University, I developed an affinity for formulas and processes. Hopefully, the RISC Analysis™ formula will help demystify the process of analyzing your contracts for you as well.

The RISC Analysis™ Defined

The RISC Analysis™ is an acronym for:
R – Reciprocity
I – Important
S – Specific
C – Customary or Standard

These four components in the RISC Analysis™ highlight the primary aspects of each term within the contract that we, as doctors, are quite capable of deciphering and understanding for ourselves. See Appendix G for your RISC Analysis™ Template.

R = RECIPROCITY

Reciprocity itself is customary and standard; it is a very common and accepted legal position and concept.

The goal of reciprocity is to achieve mutual agreement on the terms in your contract through a series of critical conversations that will take place during contract negotiations. As we will discuss extensively in Section 3, contract negotiations represent an opportunity for us to begin building a sound relationship with our future employer.

We can begin building connections by reviewing your contract through the lens of reciprocity, which respects the position of the employer while ensuring that, where applicable, the position of the employee is represented as well. This shows the prospective employer that we are knowledgeable and that we have an interest in reaching equity for both parties, where applicable. In addition, we can strategically communicate this shared goal as we work to achieve a situation where both parties are in agreement.

In the traditional sense of reciprocity, there are terms in an employment contract that should work bi-directionally in a way that is equitable to both parties. When the employer asserts for itself, then the doctor should be able to assert the same for ourselves, as well.

For example, if the employer can terminate the contract in 30 days without cause, then the doctor should also be able to terminate the contract within 30 days without cause.

On the contrary, in the sample employment agreement in Appendix T, section X reveals that the physician must give the employer 180 days' notice to terminate or renew. However, section B reveals that the employer can terminate the contract in 30 days without cause. This is not reciprocal, and this presents an opportunity for us to negotiate based on achieving reciprocity.

> *Power Move #19 - The process of negotiating our employment contract is an exercise in relationship-building. Therefore, the goal is to reach terms of mutual agreement, especially in the terms that represent your needs, aka your non-negotiables, while being communicative and collegial vs. being demanding and inflexible.*

I = IMPORTANT

As we have spent a significant amount of time in section 1 of this book, you have to identify what is important to you. Be sure that you have clarity about your needs (aka on-negotiables or deal-breakers), wants (aka negotiables), goals, objectives, and values.

Take Dr. X, for example, a newlywed who asked me to review an academic contract that she was really interested in. Once we completed our respective reviews of this document, I congratulated her on her nuptials and inquired about whether they wanted a family. "Of course!" was her response, at which time I let her know that there were no maternity leave provisions or terms specified within the contract. Well, this was certainly very important to her and ultimately constituted a deal-breaker for her and her family. However, like a boss, she was able to discuss this with the prospective employer and negotiated for maternity leave that was twice as long as the standard leave. #winning

I recommend that you have your completed Power Moves Wants and Needs Blueprint from Chapter 2 available for review before you begin analyzing your contract. This will help you focus on your priorities and prime you to look for these specifics within the terms of the contract. Reviewing with your desires in mind helps to ensure that you will start your position with a relative sense of confidence knowing that your needs and hopefully your wants will be met, or at least that they should be met according to your contract.

So, if that is maternity leave, then you want to make sure that maternity leave and the amount of maternity leave is specified in your contract; if it is a certain referral base that has been secured on your behalf to make sure you have patients coming in the door; or if it's even marketing of your arrival and opportunities for you to build a patient base—know that all of those things have to be in writing. That's a very important point.

> *Power Move #20 - If it's not in black and white →*
> *it doesn't count, and it does not have to be enforced.*

Some organizations or leadership will say, "Just trust me. You have to walk in faith, and you have to trust."

That's a big fat NO. Commitments must be documented in black and white.

> ***Power Move #21*** *- Following every negotiation conversation, always follow-up by sending the other party an email that is date and time stamped with which documents were reviewed and what was agreed upon in the conversation.*

S = SPECIFIC

Each term in your contract must be specific. Specificity in a contract refers to any term where a date, dollar figure, time frame, measurement, policy type, or data point should be indicated in that term in detail.

Specificity within a contract:

- o breeds clarity between both parties
- o adds clarity and helps us manage our expectations
- o defines the commitments and obligations that we are agreeing to
- o minimizes confusion when future situations arise, i.e., renewals or terminations
- o identifies dates and time frames
- o agree upon terms/details to be enforced
- o serves as a reference/guide for later use
- o provides protections for us professionally and personally

We need these terms in the contract to be specific so that we understand what we are committing and obligating ourselves to and that which the other party is also committing and obligating itself to.

The Opposite of Specificity

The opposite of specificity is vagueness, where quantifiable or measurable details are omitted. Such vagueness often leads to misunderstandings if any of the above issues were to arise, because the specific details are not included in the actual terms of the contract.

> Red Flag: If you have received a contract that has numerous terms that are devoid of clear definitions and other standard specifications, then this may be a Red Flag about this position and the organization.

Here are some examples that I have seen firsthand in employment contracts for doctors:

- o Malpractice insurance will be provided
- o Employee may be terminated with cause for the following reasons:
    - o excessive absenteeism
    - o chronic lateness
    - o unsatisfactory performance

These non-specific terms allow for multiple interpretations and potential understandings by the involved parties. The intent of any agreement or contract should be to elucidate and clarify each term within the contract, breeding a clear understanding by both parties.

Adding quantifiable details to the above examples of vague contract language would now look like:

- o Malpractice insurance will be provided -> Claims-made liability insurance will be provided for the doctor by the practice with limits of liability of $1,000,000/$3,000,000
- o Employee may be terminated with cause for the following reasons:

- excessive absenteeism -> absenteeism of greater than 3 continuous workdays
- chronic lateness -> reporting for one's shift more than 10 minutes late on more than X number of occasions
- unsatisfactory performance -> failing to meet baseline productivity measures of generating 20,000 RVUs annually

This second set of contract verbiage reflects a greater level of detail and specificity that we, as doctors, can certainly look for as we analyze our own contracts prior to reviewing it with our health law attorney.

Similar to studying for standardized exams or reviewing board preparatory questions, analyzing your contract for specificity is part of the review that all doctors can do because we know how to look for the quantifiable details that will help lead us to the answers.

> *Power Move #22 - Circle, highlight, or underline any vague term within the contract so that you can discuss it with your attorney before addressing it in your negotiations. This will expedite your discussion with your attorney and will empower you to be an informed client in working with them.*

This is another key reason to engage a health law attorney. While we can identify terms in general that may be vague or non-specific, your health law attorney is well-versed in the specifics of the law as it pertains to healthcare that most doctors have not been trained to identify.

C = CUSTOMARY

In addition to understanding the specifics, knowing the customary standards for the terms within a doctor's employment or other healthcare-related contract is the primary responsibility of your attorney, and this is the main reason why having a health law attorney is tantamount to your success.

Your health law attorney will interpret the legalese but will also be aware of laws and employment trends in healthcare to help build an agreement that will protect you now and throughout the term of your contract and beyond.

Just as it is our responsibility to know the ranges of normal values for CBCs, Chem 7s, and other blood work, we partner with a health lawyer who understands the standard (normal) language written into the contract that we are reviewing. We certainly would not expect our patients to know all of the parameters of normal vs. abnormal lab results. Right?

We also should not expect that while we are very smart that we would understand the legalities of state and federal regulations that are written into our contracts. We need our attorneys for this purpose.

Critical terms in the contract where customary and standard verbiage is paramount in our contracts include, but are not limited to:

- o Federal/State standards involving CMS (especially billing), HIPAA, Stark Laws, etc.
- o State licensure and reporting, which are regulations that do not allow a lot of wiggle room.
- o Credentialing
- o Malpractice Insurance, especially tail insurance, if applicable
- o Restrictive Covenants, especially Non-Compete Clauses
- o Intellectual Property
- o Referral practices
- o Practice acquisition/assumption

Partnering with a health law attorney to decipher legal compliance and possible violations of state and federal laws is one of the number one reasons that we have to partner with a health lawyer. They have a responsibility to understand the law in detail, including what is standard and customary. So, please refer back to Chapter 3 to review the questions that we should ask when interviewing health law attorneys as candidates to serve on our team of trusted advisors.

Doc: *So, what if I decide not to use an attorney to review my contract at all?*

Dr. Bonnie: *This is certainly an option, but not one that I would advise. As Attorney Kopf reminded me, most contracts include a statement that confirms that YOU have reviewed the contract in its entirety, and YOU agree to the terms therein. This essentially asserts that you are in full agreement with everything in the contract, such that you cannot claim a lack of knowledge or a lack of understanding about the contract later.*

I don't know about you, but I am not going to pretend that my medical degree has provided me with the knowledge and ability to understand EVERY aspect of an employment agreement. I've tried doing things this way, so you don't have to. Your choice!

Similarly, please refer to the sample employment agreement in Section 2 of your Power Moves Personal Workbook to practice analyzing this contract using the RISC Analysis™.

In Chapter 8, we will now apply the RISC Analysis™ as we define the most important contract terminology that every doctor should understand.

R - Reciprocal

I – Important (to me)

S - Specific

C - Customary

Figure 6 – The RISC™ Analysis Framework

NOTES

_____

_____

_____

_____

_____

_____

_____

_____

_____

_____

_____

_____

_____

_____

CHAPTER SUMMARY

POWER MOVES

- In order to build a new skill set, I recommend that every doctor read or earnestly attempt to read their own contract first, in preparation for discussing the contract with our health law attorney.
- Analyzing a contract comes after reflecting on our Power Moves Needs and Wants Blueprint.
- The process of negotiating our employment contract is an exercise in relationship-building. Therefore, the goal is to reach terms of mutual agreement, especially in the terms that represent your needs, aka your non-negotiables, while being communicative and collegial vs. being demanding and inflexible.
- Intentional Documentation from my SIP to Success Strategy™ - Following every negotiation conversation, always follow-up by sending the other party an email that is date and time stamped with which documents were reviewed and what was agreed upon in the conversation.
- Circle, highlight, or underline any vague term within the contract so that you can discuss it with your attorney before addressing it in your negotiations. This will expedite your discussion with your attorney and will empower you to be an informed client in working with them.

TAKE-HOME POINTS

- Review each term in the contract for reciprocity.
- Determine which contract terms are important to you before you begin reading the contract, then determine what is important in each term presented in the contract.
- Consult with your attorney to build your understanding of what is Customary or Standard regarding each term in your contract.
- Specificity is critical in any contract, and your employment

agreement is no different. Each term should be specific with regards to data points, dollar figures, mileage, and other quantifiable metrics, which will undoubtedly impact your ability to meet the expectations outlined in the contract. Having clarity is everything!

RED FLAGS

o   Contracts that do not reflect reciprocity and lack specificity as general principles can be concerning, and could possibly represent an organization's lack of attention to detail.

o   Now we understand that we should negotiate contract terms so that they are reciprocal and specific according to customary standards. This is so important.

o   Now that you have this knowledge, YOU (Yes, YOU) are expected to discuss and request the above during your first and second rounds of negotiations. (No worries, we will discuss this more in Chapters 10-12).

HOMEWORK

o   Hopefully, you have completed the homework from Chapter 2, and you have clarity on your needs and wants. Your goal is to first communicate these areas of critical importance to your health law attorney and other teams of advisors, then you want to make sure that these important items, which are specific to you, are accurately and specifically reflected in your contract agreement.

o   If you did not complete your <u>Power Moves Needs and Wants Blueprint</u> from Chapter 2, STOP!!! Go back and complete this exercise now, so that you can advocate for yourself by breeding clarity to your own contract negotiation.

Chapter 7

TYPES OF CONTRACTS DEFINED FOR PHYSICIANS

Doc: *This is my first year working as an independent contractor at an urgent care center. My accountant just informed me that I have to pay my own taxes and set up my own retirement and more. This is so much! Why didn't anyone tell me about this?*

Dr. Bonnie: *This can certainly be overwhelming, especially when it is unexpected. Understanding the difference between being an employee and an independent contractor is critical.*

Overview

Now that we understand a general approach as to HOW to analyze a contract, let's understand the WHAT types of contract we may encounter. The goal of this chapter is to explore how the fundamentals of the different types of contracts often correlate to the type of practice that you are going into. You will likely need to participate in an informed discussion with your attorney or other trusted advisors regarding the contract that you are reviewing.

Understanding the different types of contracts you may encounter at various stages of your career is very important because contracts contain the primary commandments of your professional and personal life.

In this chapter, we will explore the following:

- o An explanation of the options of doctor employment
- o A general overview of important salary, tax, and benefits considerations to prepare you for your conversations with your financial advisor and tax accountant
- o A detailed review of the types of contracts doctors will likely encounter

Employment Agreements (also known as Employment Contracts)

An employment agreement or contract spells out the rules of engagement between an employee and an employer. General principles that apply to most employment contracts include that:

- o The employer and an employee agree to the terms within the contract
- o It is legally enforceable, therefore, binding.
- o Compensation and expectations and benefits are typical subjects.
- o The term, i.e., the length of time of your employment, i.e., one year, is indicated.
- o The employee must agree to this contract as a condition of his/her employment.

o Employment contracts cover a variety of procedures and/or policies that are required for the employer to protect its own interest.

o The steps or consequences that will apply to either party once the employment agreement ends, based on contract expiration or termination.

As an employee, your primary responsibilities to the employer are to carry out the clinical, administrative, teaching and other duties that will be outlined in your contract. It is important to understand that your employee agreement (contract) is legally binding with consequences if either party does not fulfill the terms.

Types of Physician Employment – Employee vs. Independent Contractor

In the past ten years, trends in the doctor workforce have shifted more towards doctors moving into employed positions than in previous decades, hence the emphasis of this book on employed doctors.

One of the most common mistakes that doctors make is not understanding the difference between being an employee vs. an independent contractor and their respective benefits, tax liabilities, and financial responsibilities. Figure 7 will serve to compare and contrast these differences:

	Physician Employee	Independent Contractor
Practice Settings	• Can be employed by a hospital, university, private practice, Community-based center, MCO (i.e., Kaiser)	• Self-employed -- hospitalists, urgent care centers, emergency room settings, locums tenens
Salary & Tax Considerations	• Salary received will be your NET salary. Complete a W-4 form. • Employer is responsible for paying Tax Withholdings/ Deductions, Fed/ State Taxes, Medicare, SS (Annually or quarterly). • Employee receives a W-2 at the end of the fiscal year from the employer in order to file his/her tax return.	• Salary received will be your GROSS salary. • Complete a W-9 form. Employee is responsible for paying Tax Withholdings/DeductionsFed/ State Taxes, Medicare, SS (Annually or quarterly). • Employee receives a 1099 at the end of the fiscal year from the employer in order to file his/her tax return.
Benefits	• Benefits are customarily provided by the employer to provide benefits, re: health insurance, retirement options, etc.	• Employer does not provide benefits, re: health insurance, retirement options, etc. Malpractice insurance may or may not be covered by the employer.

Figure 7 - Employee vs. Independent Contractor Comparison Table

> Red Flag: If you are employed as an independent contractor, please note that you are responsible for obtaining your own benefits and for paying your own federal, state, FICA, and Medicare taxes. This catches many doctors off guard, so beware and be aware.

Therefore, I would advise every independent contractor to consult with a tax accountant to assist them in building a pro forma and a projected budget that will help them in calculating their federal and state tax withholdings, benefits and retirement contributions. It serves to reason that because these are significant financial considerations, I highly recommend that every doctor have their financial advisor review their contract before they sign.

Here's one last note on being an employee vs. an independent contractor. Many organizations that traditionally employ doctors as W-2 employees may also employ doctors as independent contractors as well.

Figure 8 provides an overview of the various types of practice options based on whether you are considering becoming an employed doctor, joining or starting a private practice, or practicing as an independent contractor.

Physician Employee	Independent Contractor

• Academia
  –Faculty Practice Plans
  –Physician Medical Groups
  –Medical Service Groups
• Private Practice
• Hospitals
  –Outpatient Centers
  -Hospitalists
• Community Health Center
  -Federally Qualified Health Center (FQHC)
• Managed Care Organizations (i.e., Kaiser)
• Accountable Care Organizations
	• Locums Tenens
	• Hospitalists
	• Outpatient Centers
	  -Urgent care
	  -Ambulatory centers

Figure 8 – Examples of Practice Options for Doctors

Specialty Considerations – It is important to note that doctors from all specialties can enter into any of the above practice types.

TYPES OF CONTRACTS

Considerations for New vs. Seasoned Physicians

As a new or early-career doctor, it is guaranteed that we will encounter at least 3-4 different types of contracts as we matriculate into practice. This is not even considering the types of agreements we may sign with regards to our personal lives, such as insurance, mortgages, apartment leases, automobile purchases, prenuptial agreements, etc.

Seasoned doctors, as well as new doctors for that matter, must remain aware of the constant state of change in our current healthcare environment. The corporatization of healthcare has become more prevalent in the past decade, with no signs of slowing down. Therefore, seasoned doctors will need to renegotiate for their needs and wants when renewing their employment contracts. Whereas employment contracts in the 1990s and early 2000s were more doctor friendly, one cannot assume that a renewal contract even from the same institution will be as doctor friendly as it may have once been.

Contracts for Doctors in Training – Residency and Fellowship Contracts

Residency Contracts

One of the initial contracts that you will encounter as a young doctor will be a residency employment contract, in which you will be an employee of the hospital or medical center. The residency contract is an employment agreement between you and the training institution where you have matched. As such, all of the rights and benefits that are afforded to every hospital employee also apply to you as a resident, such as the following:

It is important that you review your residency contract, not just for the compensation from a benefits perspective. As a hospital employee, you can likely begin saving for retirement even in residency as a part of any retirement savings plan that the hospital has set up for its body of employees. Check with your human resources department and confer with your financial advisor to discuss this option during training.

Also, your residency contract is likely the last contract that you will sign that has a guaranteed number of terms that are written to support you as the resident. This will be the last contract that does so by default, as residency contracts have to abide by the institution's policies and regulations in order for training programs to remain credentialed.

Most residents do not obtain an attorney to review their contracts. However, it is very important that you obtain a copy of your signed contract once it has been signed by both parties, i.e., executed.

One additional note: Please investigate whether you will be training in a state in which residents are part of a union, and unionized employees have contractual protections that are conferred through their union membership.

Fellowship Contracts

Depending on whether a particular fellowship is an accredited fellowship training program or not, your contract may address your employment as a fellow to reflect the stipulations that apply to attending doctors versus that of resident trainees. In fact, some fellowship agreements include restrictive covenants such as non-compete clauses. Therefore, a careful review of one's fellowship contract is certainly warranted. I have seen some fellowship contracts include non-compete clauses, so be careful to review these contracts carefully, especially if you are considering practicing in the same region in which your fellowship is located.

Contracts for Doctors in Practice

First & Second Employment Contracts for Doctors – The Process

For doctors entering employed practices with compensation models that are based on productivity or if partnership opportunities exist, it is important to understand the most common process for employing doctors in these situations.

(NOTE: The following information applies to doctors entering medical practices as employees, excluding those entering large managed care organizations, e.g., Kaiser.)

Commonly, doctors will encounter a series of two contracts when joining a new practice:

- o The initial contract, which I refer to as a Foundation Agreement (Contract)
- o The second contract, which I refer to as the Renewal Agreement (Contract)

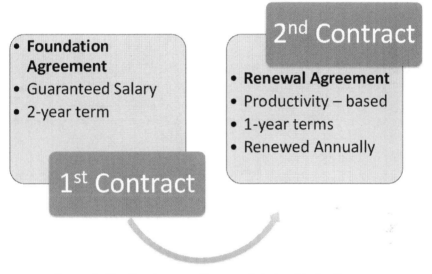

Figure 9 - The Employment Contract Relationship for Doctors

The Foundation Agreement

I describe the first contract in this series as the Foundation Agreement, because this contract will provide you with a financial foundation, if managed correctly. This first contract, or Foundation Agreement, should reflect the compensation that is customary or standard within the norm of your specialty in your particular geographic region.

An additional point about your first Foundation Contract is that this agreement will span the doctor's initial term, usually 1-2 years in practice, and it customarily provides the doctor with a guaranteed annual salary that is NOT BASED ON PRODUCTIVITY.

Why? Practices understand that it takes 12-24 months for doctors who are new to a practice to understand, then increase their workflow efficiency, to build a patient base, and to become familiar with coding and billing. In addition, if we think about it, as a doctor that is new to any practice, every patient seen will be a new patient to the new doctor, even if the patient is an established patient in the practice. After all, we know that more time is required to see new patients than established ones, so this first contract allows for this increased time requirement while decreasing the pressure to productivity requirements while ramping up one's practice.

At the time of publishing of this book, most compensation models for employed physicians are based on a productivity model (see Bonus Chapter 9 for more details), doctors will engage in a series of two contracts with a practice. This is based on the assumption that the doctor renews their contract with the employer at the end of their first term.

While this Foundation Agreement provides some initial financial stability for the doctor, please know that your productivity is being monitored and documented by the practice. Why? Because in this Foundation Agreement, which likely spans years 1 and 2, the standard holds that your compensation in year 3 will be based on your productivity in year 2. Get it? The productivity expectation for your initial term of the practice is that in:

o   Year 1 - Doctor becomes familiar with the practice dynamics with a slow increase in the number of patients the doctor sees over that year
o   Year 2 - The number of patients seen increases to a level that has stabilized or continues to grow

o Year 3 – Should the doctor decide to renew their contract with this practice, the doctor's Year 3 compensation will be based on their previous performance in year 2, usually within a specific time interval.

> ***Power Move #23*** *- Do your due diligence on the fair market value for compensation norms for your specialty, in your specific region and practice type. Don't forget to work your network of colleagues who have recently transitioned into the workforce.*

For the sake of simplicity, Figure 10 demonstrates the flow and differentiates between the Foundation Agreement and the Renewal Agreement.

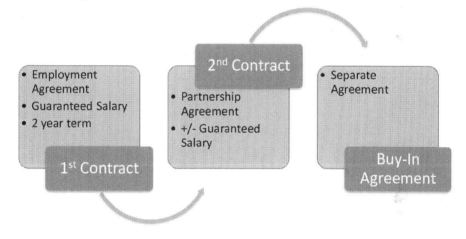

Figure 10 - The Employment Contract Relationship for Doctors

The Renewal Agreement

This second contract, the Renewal Agreement, can actually be thought of as the most important agreement of the two because this is the agreement that will dictate how you will be compensated based on productivity. It will also specify any additional means for compensation moving forward. Why is this so important? Because when we do not understand the level of variability that can occur in a practice's billing, collections, and documentation routines, it can cost us thousands of dollars in lost, uncollected, or undocumented revenue.

I cannot tell you how many doctors call me every year to say that their practice has just notified them that they will be receiving, for example, a 25% pay cut, or a $100,000 decrease in their annual salary. The practice likely notes that in the previous year, or other designated time period, that the doctor's productivity was not high enough to maintain their previous salary.

Well, this may or may not be true. As part of our SIP to SUCCESS theory, the "I" encourages us to be intentional with our documentation. It is inordinately critical that each doctor documents and keeps a copy of our own productivity in every setting, which should include any consults, add-ons, or other non-scheduled patients that will contribute to productivity calculations. Do not count on "Ms. Doe" the office manager, to keep an accounting of your productivity

> *Power Move #24* - *ALWAYS keep your own documentation on the numbers, diagnoses, and procedures. (After all, we documented our patients and cases in residency, so let's just keep it going.)*

In addition, it is important we build relationships with the doctor leaders and business administrators in the group so that you can review how your productivity is being monitored and calculated, usually on an RVU model. Again, it does not benefit the collections staff members, who receive a steady salary that is not based on productivity, to accurately document and tabulate your productivity for you. This is up to you, and you can have to request to meet with the administrators at least on a monthly basis so that the two of you can compare your data and RVU calculations to ensure accuracy.

Employment Contract Exceptions

This information applies to doctors entering medical practices as employees, excluding those entering large managed care organizations, such as Kaiser and others, which do not routinely or may only minimally be willing to negotiate with their prospective employees.

Doctors Entering Private Practice & Buy-Ins

Similar to the doctors in the previous section, for doctors joining a private practice, the process customarily holds that the doctor will sign an employment agreement for an initial term.

For those doctors who are joining a private practice, one of the first questions that should be asked is whether becoming a partner or shareholder in the practice is an option. It is important that you want to understand what is expected in order to achieve partnership. The following types of questions should be asked:

- o What is the time frame designated in order to achieve partnership?
- o What are the eligibility qualifications for becoming a partner?
- o Is there an equity buy-in that is required? Meaning, are you required to buy shares of equity of the organization in the organization that you are becoming a part of?
- o Are buy-outs part of the partnership agreement, and if so, what is the formula that will be used?

Additional questions that should be asked include[4]:

- o What is the total compensation expected each year until partnership (i.e., understanding levels of incentive compensation and the likelihood of payment)?
- o What is the partnership buy-in structure?
- o Are all partners treated equally, or does a 1 or 2 tier partnership system exist?

o How many doctors/partners have left in the past 3 years? For what reasons?

These are important questions to ask because during your first contract term with the practice as an employee, you will be assessing the practice to see whether this practice is a good fit for you to join as a partner. In other words, your first two years in the practice will be the time period during which you are dating. Bi-directionally you and the practice are determining whether either party wants to move forward to partnership, which is just like a marriage, by the way.

> Red Flag: If practices are unwilling to share or are unclear about the pathway to partnership, view this as a Red Flag. Due to the gravity that partnership, which makes you part owner of the practice, holds, clarity regarding the business, legal, and financial obligations required to become and to remain a partner should be made very clear to you in understandable terms so that you have full knowledge to base your decision on.

Once you have met the eligibility requirements and your partnership has been approved by the current practice leadership, a partnership agreement will be signed by both you and your partners. This agreement will outline the rights of each partner in the practice and will determine how you and your partners will address decisions that affect the practice as a whole. It will discuss the practice's obligations to you as a partner, as well as your obligations to the practice. It will also address details of dissolution, in case, for some reason, you no longer wish to be a partner in that practice.

Keep in mind that just because partnership is being offered does not mean that you have to accept the offer, especially if your first contract term as an employee reveals aspects of the practice that would dissuade you from wanting to become an owner. Contrastingly, partnership offers financial upsides if the practice is profitable, in addition to other benefits of partnership that the practice should outline to potential future partners.

To review the process for joining a private practice with a partnership track or ownership/shareholder option, here are the chronological steps:

o Year 1 – Physician becomes familiar with the practice dynamics with a slow increase in the number of patients the doctor sees over that year.

o Year 2 – The number of patients seen increases to a level that has stabilized or continues to grow. The physician works to satisfy the requirements for partnership. Both partners observe the other party to assess fit for partnership.

o Year 3 or more – Once partnership has been offered to the doctor, a separate partnership agreement should be extended to the doctor from the practice detailing the practice's obligations to the partner and vice versa.

o Year 3 – An additional buy-in agreement may be presented for signature because this agreement will specify the financial investment, if any, required from the doctor in order to buy-in to the practice's equity.

Even at the time that your initial employment contract is signed, not the amount, but how the buy-in calculated should be reviewed with you in lieu of a dollar figure.

Once you have satisfied the terms of your initial agreement, making you eligible to buy into the equity of the practice, the buy-in agreement outlines exactly what aspects of the practice you are buying into, how much it will cost, the buy-in, and how the buy-in will be transacted. It is important to make sure that you are buying into the assets with value that the company owns and that you are not just purchasing goodwill, or invisible assets. Assets with value that are owned by the practice include its accounts receivable, any real estate, ancillary services, hardware, or equipment.

> *Power Move #25* - *Make sure you understand the buy-in calculation and/or the additional partnership eligibility requirements at the time that you sign the first employment agreement with the private practice.*

An additional component of a partnership agreement is the buy-out arrangement that may apply if one of the partners in the group decides to leave or retire from the practice and will no longer be an owner, essentially dissolving their equity stake in the practice. In a buy-out, the remaining partners agree to literally buy back the amount of the practice's equity from the departing partner. Similarly, a buy-out agreement will outline exactly how much it will cost to buy, how to affect the buy-out, and how the buy-out will be transacted. This could amount to significant financial outlay from each partner, especially if a senior partner retires shortly after you become a partner. Thus, it is important for potential partners to ask about the prospects of any of the senior partners retiring or if there are other potential corporate changes pending.

> *Power Move #26* - *Ask as many questions as possible to assess the culture, fit, financial management, strategy, and plans, i.e., mergers, acquisitions, departures, or purchases, BEFORE signing on as a partner.*

So, these are some of the key elements that you will find in a partnership agreement. However, it is important to know as well that, even if you are joining a practice in which partnership is an option, you do not have to take the partnership track, and you do not have to become a partner. You can remain an employee if that is your goal. But the requirements for becoming a partner should be spelled out early and very clearly.

Additional Contract Types for Doctors in Private Practice – Leases for Property or Medical Equipment

An additional lease agreement that doctors in private practice would likely encounter is an office lease, which is usually a commercial real estate lease that is uniquely different from residential leases. Commercial leases usually have an extended term of a minimum of five years and can extend up to ten years or more. It is important to note the length of time required or expounded upon in this office lease so that the practice understands the amount of time that it is committing to rent this same office space. Also in a commercial lease, there will be CAM (common area maintenance) cost, and there will also be stipulations regarding utilities, signage, parking, disposal of hazardous waste, the cost of any repairs, system malfunctions such as the commercial heating or air conditioning units. Failure to do our due diligence regarding commercial leases can prove to be extremely costly if we are not clear and careful about what we are signing. So please take the time to speak with an advisor, perhaps even a commercial realtor or real estate attorney, who has experience in reviewing a commercial real estate lease so that you can ensure that you are signing a lease that is compatible with the type of practice that you want.

Also, in private practice, one might encounter the acquisition of equipment either via purchase or leases. Most equipment lease agreements will allow you to rent equipment from the company that owns the equipment. Because medical equipment is usually costly, equipment leases will allow the lessee, i.e., the practice, to pay an agreed-upon monthly rental fee with an interest rate attached.

As a partner or part owner, the doctor will likely have to sign a lease agreement, which means you and the practice are committing and obligating yourself to making the lease payments, the equipment lease payments, during the term of the agreement, the length of time of the agreement, for the indicated amount that has to be paid, by the monthly due date.

Personal Loan Guarantees

Important: Equipment leases require some form of guarantee or collateral to ensure that the practice will make the required payments. Especially for smaller private practices, the lessor many times requires that the doctors PERSONALLY GUARANTEE that the monthly payments will be made when one personally guarantees a lease or loan of any type. That means not only is the practice liable and responsible to make sure that the monthly payments are made on time, but it also means that the doctor as an individual is now essentially leveraging his or her own assets and making them accessible to the bank as collateral in case any damages done to the equipment or in case the payments are not made on a timely basis.

This is a very important concept and a potential landmine. A personal guarantee for any loan means that your individual assets can be levied to cover the payment on the lease or the outstanding loan. If that lease or loan goes into default, meaning the lease or loan payments are not paid, your assets can be accessed as collateral payment for the outstanding dollar amounts owed.

Doctors Entering Academia

Many academic contracts will be presented to you as a new faculty member in two parts.

The first part of the academic contract is usually the letter of intent, also called a commitment letter or term sheet, which should be issued by the department chair of the academic department. The letter of intent is usually two to three pages in length and primarily outlines the following terms within the contract:

- o Proposed academic title (which is negotiable)
- o Term (length) of the contract
- o Duties and responsibilities associated with this position, which would include your clinical research, teaching, and/or administration administrative duties. These duties would be outlined in the form of a percentage or in the form of percentages.
    - o For example, your duties might be 70% clinical, 10%

        research, 10% teaching, and 10% administrative or leadership compensation would also be addressed in this letter of intent.
- o On-call coverage
- o Compensation and the model by which the compensation will be calculated. The institutional parties that are responsible for each component of your compensation should be detailed as well.
  - o Using the example above, if 70% of your time will be spent performing clinical activities, then the hospital or medical center will likely support 70% of your salary and the remaining 30% for your research, teaching and administrative duties collectively may be paid for by the hospital's affiliated medical school.
- o Locations of your clinical and teaching duties
- o Any other specifics that you have negotiated with your department chair or Dean should be outlined in this term letter.

This letter of intent or term letter is presented separately to the individual doctor because it contains the specific details of the contract that were negotiated between the doctor and the department. These are the details that can vary between doctors, and therefore each doctor will receive a customized term letter once negotiations have ended.

The second part of an academic contract usually consists of the standard employee handbook for all of the institution's faculty. This handbook outlines the non-negotiable details the rules and regulations that apply to all employees and faculty throughout the institution, such as:

- o Benefits packages, including
  - o Health, dental, and vision insurance policy options
  - o Retirement/savings plan participation
  - o Leave for illness, personal time, and continuing medical education (CME)
- o Promotions packet, which gives the details and definitions of each academic position title and the scholarly criteria for

every academic title in the institution. Requirements for promotion to an advanced level are included in the Promotions packet as well.

So, in academia, you can see that you are looking at a two-part agreement, and you will need to make sure that you have thoroughly reviewed each component of that agreement prior to signing. Again, we will not assume that because our chairperson or leadership really like us, that this contract is inclusive of our wants and needs. Again, it is up to us to negotiate even in an academic contract where these contracts are traditionally less likely to be negotiated.

However, this trend is changing with the corporatization of medicine, many academic departments have now morphed into various permutations of independent practices, such as faculty practice plans, doctor medical groups, and medical service groups.

Finally, for those entering Academia, please refer to the most comprehensive reference available, Succeeding in Academia, by Dr. John Sanchez (Ed.) et al[5]. This reference text describes in necessary detail every aspect of transitioning into and succeeding in an academic practice.

(Full Disclosure: I am a co-author of the chapter entitled, "Finding an Academic Position" in Succeeding in Academia. I do not receive any monetary gain from the sale of this textbook.)

Independent Contractor Agreements

The next type of contract is the independent contractor agreement.

Any doctor who is providing services as an independent contractor should know that the employer is not responsible for withholding your federal, state, or FICA taxes. This is the responsibility of the independent contractor. That's you! Therefore, independent contractor compensation rates might be able to be negotiated to be a somewhat higher level.

As noted previously in this chapter, you are required to make your own estimated tax payments, and I highly recommend that every independent contractor discuss the tax implications and build a tax strategy with your accountant prior to signing any contract.

> ***Power Move #27*** *- As part of your due diligence, have your tax accountant, in addition to your health law attorney and your financial advisor, review your contract BEFORE signing on the dotted line.*

Additional responsibilities that independent contractors will need to address include acquiring and covering the costs of:

- o Benefits packages, including
  - o Health, dental, and vision insurance policy options
  - o Retirement/savings plan participation
  - o Leave for illness, personal time, and continuing medical education (CME)
- o Malpractice insurance (in some cases)

You have to be increasingly aware and astute of these expenses that will not be withheld from your paycheck as they would if you were an employee. It is even more critical for independent contractors to have their team of trusted advisors intact so that from the very beginning, you can address your tax obligations as well as make sure that your benefits and protections are in place.

Please see the section on Employment in Chapter 8 on Contract Terms for additional details regarding independent contractors.

Locum Tenens Contracts
Locum Tenens, which means in Latin to hold a place for, is a temporary type of employment for doctors that allows for practices to hire doctors temporarily to fill a needed position.

Due to the temporary nature of this position, most locum tenens contracts are independent contractor agreements or contracts, which will require that the doctor makes our own tax payments and secures our own benefits in most cases. However, these contracts are highly negotiable; therefore, it is imperative that doctors confer with other doctors who have extensive locum tenens experience. I personally recommend Dr. Stephanie Freeman, who actually has an online course for doctors who are interested in learning more about locum tenens as an employment option.

Other Types of Contracts Doctors are Likely to Encounter

Payer-Provider Agreements

If you are practicing medicine in a practice that participates in the third-party reimbursement system, you will, as an individual doctor, likely be required to sign a payer-provider agreement.

This is a contract between you as the doctor and your NPI and the third-party insurer, such as Aetna, Cigna, Blue Cross Blue Shield, etc., indicating that you agree to be listed as a provider on their panel for patients to choose from, and you are also agreeing to accept the reimbursement rates offered in the agreement.

Exceptions:

- o   If you are working for an organization that is self-insured, such as Kaiser, then you will not need to sign payor-provider agreements, because Kaiser is self-insured.
- o   Cash pay, such as concierge, practices, or direct primary care practices, are other examples of practices that do not participate in the third-party payer system, and therefore payer-provider agreements are not signed in these practices.

More specifically, if your organization bills the Centers for Medicare and Medicaid Services (CMS), Blue Cross Blue Shield, or any of the other commercial payers, you are almost guaranteed to be required to sign your own individual payer-provider agreement.

Because most practices see patients or enroll patients from several insurers' panels, you will likely have to sign a separate payer-provider agreement for each insurance company that your practice works with.

It is critical, especially in small to midsize practices, that the billing and collections department in your practice keeps a copy of the payer-provider agreements that each doctor has signed. Each payer-provider agreement will outline renewal dates and the negotiated reimbursement rates for every billing code on a fee schedule.

It is extremely critical that those payer-provider agreements be monitored on an annual basis, as the fee schedule can be reviewed and actually negotiated such that you can, in your practice, negotiate for higher reimbursement rates with that particular insurance company. Re-negotiation of reimbursement rates is not always successful, but it is detrimental to the practice if upon evaluating an insurance company's reimbursement rates, the practice finds that it can no longer cover its overhead costs due to low reimbursements. Practices then have a tough choice to make a) see more patients or b) choose not to be on that insurer's provider panel.

Insurance Policies are Contracts, too!

An additional subset of contracts includes the various types of insurance policies including,

- o Malpractice
- o Life
- o Disability
- o Long-term care

These types of insurance can be categorized under a general umbrella of income protection policies that are secured via a contract between you, the beneficiary, and the policyholder, i.e., the insurance company.

In this contract, you agree to pay a monthly amount, called a premium, in order to secure insurance protection, in-case of loss of life, ability to practice, or other benefits and changes. In exchange, the insurance company has specific criteria outlined in your policy, i.e., your contract, which dictates the terms under which you will receive the insurance protection if you were to file a claim. Therefore, it is VERY important that you understand the terms of the policy, especially when it comes to your malpractice and disability insurance policies.

> *Power Move #28* - *Review the terms of your insurance policies with your insurance broker, who may be your financial advisor, on an annual basis, or when major life events/transitions happen in your life.*

Obtaining insurance protection is, in fact, a process.

- o Once you apply for the specific type of insurance, the insurance company will decide whether they are going to underwrite, i.e., approve your policy.
    - o Additional information or evaluations may be required if the underwriters do not initially approve your policy
    - o It is customary for insurance companies to require a health evaluation if you are over a specific age or if you have pre-existing health conditions, especially when applying for life or disability insurance
- o Once the underwriters have approved your application, you will sign the policy in order to bind insurance protection from that company.

> **Power Move #29** - It is up to you to obtain copies of your own insurance policies and keep them in a secure digital file, as well as a hard copy, which should be kept in a fire-proof, waterproof safe. (See Appendix D & E for my Master Organization List of Documents that every doctor must have at their fingertips.)

Promissory Notes and your Signing Bonus – Landmine Alert

The final contract that we will review is called a promissory note or agreement one signs when securing or taking out a loan. This note represents the promise of one party to repay the loan provider within a certain term, length of time, and interest rate.

Doc, here is why this is important to us. Many doctor employers, hospitals, academic centers, and private practices are now offering signing or relocation "bonuses" and other compensation in the form of a reimbursable loan, which is usually unclear to the doctor. In addition to the "Bonus" terminology being misleading, the terms, i.e., the details regarding repayment of the loan, may also be unfavorable.

For example:

> Dr. B is offered a $36,000 signing "bonus" in the initial contract offer. Dr. B is excited about this access to cash and signs the Promissory Note found in Appendix A, of the contract. Important note: The term of Dr. B's employment contract is for 2 years.

> At 18 months into his contract, Dr. B gets engaged and does not want to renew his contract in 6 months. Unfortunately, Dr. B was unaware that his signing bonus was actually a loan, that has a 3-year monthly loan repayment term with an interest rate of prime + 1%.

Interpretation: When Dr. B accepted the $36,000 at the beginning of his employment term, he agreed to have a specific amount deducted from his paycheck monthly to repay the loan at an interest rate that is higher than the "prime" interest rate generally charged by banks. #yikes

However, the promissory note also indicated that the term of the repayment was over a 3-year period, although the term of his employment was over a 2-year period.

Unfortunately for young Dr. B, this means that if he does not renew his contract at the end of his first 2 year term, that he will have to pay back the balance of the loan at an interest rate of prime + 1%. In other words, hopefully Dr. B did not spend the entirety of the initial $36,000 signing "bonus" amount, because he will now need to write a check for approximately $12,000 + interest owed.

Dr. B does have the option of renewing his contract for one additional year in order to complete the repayment of the loan amount, which means he will not be moving to be with his fiancée at this time.

In the end, Dr. B wrote the practice a check for the balance owed, and he did move to be with his fiancée. However, they had to delay their wedding in order to build up their cash savings prior to getting married at the advice of their financial advisor.

This is a key example of how our contract can affect not only our professional life but our personal lives and financial stability.

Specific caution lies in the fact that some doctors are already saddled with a significant amount of educational loan debt. It is imperative for each doctor to assess if additional loan amounts offered by the organization or employer are critical to their existence or not.

Certainly, a young doctor might agree to accept a "bonus" when signing or relocating for a new position, but would the same new doctor agree to take on an additional amount of loan debt in order to have access to cash at the beginning of their professional career? Maybe or maybe not, but having the loan disguised as a loan is, in fact, a deceptive practice that I have seen written into contracts more and more frequently in recent years.

We have a choice as to whether we signed on for these additional amounts of cash given our financial status or state once we have moved into practice as we move into practice.

This is why it is critically important that every doctor does their due diligence by having our contracts reviewed by a trusted advisor, preferably our accountant and financial advisor, possibly even our banker, so that these trusted advisors can weigh in on the full gamut of financial and tax ramifications that are associated with this contract so that we understand upfront what we are walking into.

> *Power Move #30 - Take caution and time to do your due diligence when it comes to signing any contract.*

Conclusion - Here's How to Apply the "SIP to Success" Theory to Any Contract

It is our obligation to be more strategic when we are signing our employment agreements or any other type of contract.

Therefore, it is critically important that we not sign any contract expeditiously, although we may be being pressured to do so from the organization or from their representative.

It is virtually impossible to have all of your trusted advisors review and weigh in on your contract within a 5-7 day period of time, the time frame that many recruiters and potential employers will give a doctor to review their contract. It is reasonable for you to request at least 30 days for you to review the contract agreement with your advisors in doing your due diligence.

This is a reasonable request and my recommended approach with sample language:

"Thank you so much for sending over this agreement. I have received your request to have it signed and returned to you within the next 5-7 business days. However, I would like to respectfully request additional time to review this agreement with my advisors as part of my due diligence. Certainly, you understand that I want to make the best, most informed decisions in order to achieve a win-win for both me and you, as my potential employer. I will make sure to get back to you with my initial questions in the next 10-20 business days. I remain excited about this offer."

Ideally, you should proactively communicate this response verbally, preferably via phone, then you MUST follow-up your conversation with an email, documenting with intention the above and any other details from your conversation with the potential employer.

> **Red Flag:** If an organization does not agree to allow you to have time to do your due diligence, which includes having time to review your agreement with your advisory team to enable you to make the best decision for yourself and your family, then you have to be prepared to walk away. If they are not willing to accommodate more time for you to make an educated assessment of your contract, then this is an indication and a Red Flag that this may not be a doctor friendly environment

It is customary and standard for contract reviews and negotiations to take 30, 60, and sometimes 90 days such that both parties have all of their questions answered, reaching a consensus and achieving an employment position and contract everyone involved feels good about.

> *Power Move #31 - We do NOT make six-figure decisions in a five-day period of time!*

CHAPTER SUMMARY

POWER MOVES

- o Do your due diligence on the fair market value for compensation norms for your specialty, in your specific region and practice type.
- o ALWAYS keep your own documentation on the numbers, diagnoses, and procedures.
- o Make sure you understand the buy-in calculation and/or the additional partnership eligibility requirements at the time that you sign the first employment agreement with the private practice.
- o Ask as many questions as possible to assess the culture, fit, financial management, strategy, and plans, i.e., mergers, acquisitions, departures, or purchases BEFORE signing on as a partner.
- o As part of your due diligence, have your tax accountant, in addition to your health law attorney and your financial advisor, review your contract BEFORE signing on the dotted line.
- o Take caution and time to do your due diligence when it comes to signing any contract.
- o We do NOT make six-figure decisions in a five-day period of time!

RED FLAGS

- o If practices are unwilling to share or are unclear about the pathway to partnership,
- o If an organization does not agree to allow you to have time to do your due diligence

HOMEWORK

- o Review the terms of your insurance policies with your insurance broker, who may be your financial advisor, on an annual basis, or when major life events/transitions happen in your life.

o It is up to you to obtain copies of your own insurance policies and keep them in a secure digital file, as well as a hard copy, which should be kept in a fire-proof, waterproof safe.

REFERENCES

4. Mason BS, Boike, K, Haas, R. "The Art of Renegotiation." Chicago Medicine Magazine, September 2016.

5. Sanchez, John P. (Ed.) Succeeding in Academic Medicine - a Roadmap for Diverse Medical Students and Residents. Springer. 978-3-030-33266-2, 489284_1_En, (4).

NOTES

_____

_____

_____

_____

_____

_____

_____

_____

_____

_____

_____

_____

_____

Chapter 8

CONTRACT TERMINOLOGY

Doc: *What does all of this $#$% (contract language) mean, and why should I care?*

Dr. Bonnie: *Because your life depends on it.*

The goal of this chapter is to provide definitions of the common employment contract terms in an easily digestible fashion due to the current trend of physicians electing to transition into employed physicians[4].

How to Use this Chapter

Because of the quantity of content in this chapter, I recommend reviewing this one term at a time in order to:

o build a better understanding of the critical elements of an employment contract

o identify details in each contract term that are specific to your specialty that are not included in this general discussion

o understand the numerous variations that can apply to each term

o share learned experiences from other doctors regarding each term

o prevent becoming overwhelmed

In this chapter, we will review the terms according to the anatomical comparisons used in Chapter 5:

o The Face - which describes the opening paragraph containing critical definitions that will be referenced throughout the contract

o The Body - which describes the most important terms of the contract, including the Top 5 contract terms that all doctors should understand

o The Extremities - which refers to the compensation and the specific compensation model being offered will be discussed in Chapter 9

CONTRACT COMMONALITIES

The core of most contracts contains the same or similar fundamental terms. This content is usually broken up into headings, which can include definitions, terms, exhibits, and appendices. However, do not rely on headings only for what's in the paragraph. Other things can be hidden. Read it all (or something like that in your words)

In every well-formatted employment contract, there are approximately 15 terms that I highly recommend every doctor become familiar with. Though not always organized in a particular order, understanding these terms will enable doctors to:

- know the core components of most contracts and
- have an informed conversation with your attorney and other trusted advisors regarding the contract
- avoid some of the most common professional and financial landmines and mistakes that doctors have made in my experience

Here are the 15 contract terms for doctors to understand.

- Term and Termination*
- Professional Liability (Malpractice) Insurance*
- Covenant Not to Compete*
- Intellectual Property/Outside Revenue*
- Definitions
- Employment
- Duties and Responsibilities
- Effects of Termination
- Non-Disclosure/Non-Solicitation
- Ownership Opportunity
- Compensation
  - Salary
    - Base Pay
    - Variable Pay
- Fringe Benefits*
- Leave – Education, Vacation, Sick, Personal time
- Relocation Expenses

This list of contract terms can serve as your primary checklist when reviewing a contract. Please see The Doctor's Ultimate Guide to Contracts and Negotiations Workbook #2 for a blank Contract

Terminology Checklist to be used when negotiating your next contract. The "Top 5 Most Important Contract Terms" are those marked with an asterisk, as these are terms that can result in negative consequences, even more so than our compensation.

> Red Flag: Experience has taught me to read the entire contract because important information may be buried in different sections of the contract. For example, specifics about tail insurance may appear in other parts of the contract, such as in the Termination or Effects of Termination sections, and not just in the section on malpractice insurance.

> *Power Move #32 - Always review these Top 5 Contract Terms in every contract:*
> *Term and Termination*
> *Non-compete Clause*
> *Malpractice Insurance*
> *Intellectual Property/ Outside Revenue Generation*
> *Fringe Benefits*

We will define the terms of the contract using a case scenario describing employment contracts offered to a young doctor seeking to find her first position after residency. Her name is C. A. Doctor, M.D., and she is a primary care doctor who is completing a fellowship in non-invasive cardiology. For now, pay special attention to these Top 5 Terms that I recommend all doctors become familiar with.

EXPLORING CONTRACT TERMINOLOGY

The Face – The Opening Paragraph

Doc: *I was assured that I would be working solely out of the practice location that is closest to my home. Now, I am being required to take on-call duties at a hospital that is two hours away from my home without traffic. Please advise.*

Dr. Bonnie: *Before signing your contract, please take the time to literally map out each practice location on a map to understand the scope of the practice's geographic reach, which should be referred to in this opening paragraph. Then, negotiate to have your location preferences reflected in the contract.*

Note: With the acceleration of practice acquisitions by large hospital systems, our health law attorney can best help us negotiate terms regarding the reassignment of doctors to new practice sites in the future, as in this case above.

The first paragraph of the contract, the face, identifies and defines the who, when, and where of the contract.

Core Concepts: Specifically identified are the parties who are engaging in a relationship to exchange something of value, such as exchanging financial compensation for healthcare services rendered by the physician. This paragraph will also define how the parties will be addressed throughout the agreement, for example:

- o   The hospital system will be referred to as the "Employer"
- o   C. A. Doctor, MD will be referred to as the "Employee"

In addition, the corporate status of both parties, the state of employment, and the date of the contract are identified as well. Essentially, these key definitions which will identify:

- o   Who – names the parties who are engaging in this business arrangement?
  - o The prospective employer
    - ▪ the name of employer, medical center, hospital
    - ▪ its corporate status, i.e., Professional Corporation (PC), Not-for-Profit organization (NFP)
    - ▪ and subsidiaries or satellites

o the prospective employee, i.e., the physician
- o When – The initial date of the contract offers and the expected employment work date
- o Where – Relevant practice locations
- o What – Type of employment may be referenced

Referring back to this section frequently while reviewing your contract for clarification of definitions is highly recommended, it is best to spend a few minutes initially familiarizing yourself with this section from the start.

So, what is important? Let's use the RISC Analysis to find out.

- o Reciprocity – Both parties, their corporate structure and the states in which their companies operate should be listed, including that of the doctor who may or may not have their own LLC or S-Corp as an independent contractor.
- o Important – The opening paragraph will identify subsidiaries and satellite office locations for a practice or hospital system. Identifying this information will be helpful when reviewing the non-compete clause later in the contract.
- o Specific – Being assigned or reassigned to multiple clinical locations can be disruptive to our professional and personal lives. Be sure to inquire about this specifically. Be sure to get clarity about the addresses of the locations of these satellites and whether you will be assigned to work at multiple satellite locations, then use Intentional Documentation to ensure that your location assignments are reflected in your final contract before signing.
- o Customary – These terms should be in the opening paragraphs and are standard in every type of contract.

Defining Terms in the Body of the Contract

TERM (i.e., the LENGTH of the contract)

Doc: Dr. Bonnie, my contract has a start date but not an end date. Is that a problem?

Dr. Bonnie: *Not only is this a problem, but this is a contract that could run into perpetuity, i.e., forever, which does not give us a renewal nor expiration date around which we can renegotiate the terms of our contract in the future. Yes, we must know the start and end dates of the agreement.*

Core Concepts: This term specifies the length of your contractual obligation. Be sure to check the dates of the initial length of the contract. Further employment options, i.e., renewals, expirations, and terminations, should be found here.

The renewal or non-renewals, i.e., explanation expiration date of the contract is important. This term will indicate the amount of time that you will have to give notice to either renew the contract or to indicate that you will not renew the contract, i.e., that you intend to let it expire.

So, what is important here? Let's use the RISC Analysis to find out.

- o   Reciprocity – This term of the contract should specify the start and end (expiration or renewal) dates of the term of the contract.
- o   Important – Knowing the dates of your renewal/re-negotiation window is critical because timing is everything. The initial term of the contract may be different than the renewal term (length) of the contract, which often corresponds to a shift in the compensation model being offered.
- o   Specific – Specific dates for the start and termination/expiration and renewal of the contract should be provided.
- o   Customary – This is standard information that should be present in every contract, please look for it and make sure that you know what you are signing up for.

> Red Flag – The actual length or term of the contract indicated in this section of the contract can sometimes be overridden based on the termination without cause term of the contract. (If this sounds like I am speaking a foreign language, rest assured that we will cover this next in the Termination section.)

TERMINATION:

Doc: I can't believe it. I was just fired...for no clear reason. I didn't know this could happen. How is this possible?

Dr. Bonnie: How one gets out of a contract is just as important as how you get into the contract! Most often, we pay closer attention to how we transition into a practice while omitting the details around how this professional relationship could end.

Core Concepts: The **termination** clause goes hand in hand with the term (length of contract) clause. Termination identifies the circumstances around which your employment can be terminated by the employer,

with or without cause, i.e., with or without a reason.

In other words, the termination clause outlines the employer's exit strategy for ending the contract for your employment prior to the end of the contract's term, as they deem necessary. (The good news is that it can outline your exit strategy as well.)

With or without cause means that the employer can give you a reason for terminating you, i.e., with cause, OR the employer can terminate you without giving you a reason, i.e., without cause.

Though this may not seem fair, the good news is that this term in your contract should be reciprocal such that you, the doctor, can also exercise your right to terminate your contract with or without cause.

Thus, you must identify the separate clause that allows you to terminate without cause. Usually for an employee to terminate with cause, there has to be a breach of something material, i.e., important, by the employer, such as not paying you.

Termination (with or without cause) clauses usually require:

○ a specific and detailed list of all of the "for cause" reasons that the doctor may be terminated. Make sure that you read and understand each of these "for cause" reasons. Ask for clarity if you do not understand these reasons, if they are vague or non-specific.

○ an opportunity for the receiving party to "cure," i.e., fix the problem or address the reason for the other party's termination

○ the terminating party notifies the other party in writing within a specified number of days.

○ the number of days required for giving the other party notice of termination should be approximately close, if not equal, for both the employer and the employee.

○ Exception - Because the employer has to avoid patient abandonment claims, the employer may request a greater number of days' notice from the employee.

Red Flag Example: I have read an employment contract where the employer indicated that the employee provided 180 days written notice, but the employer could give the employee 30 days' written notice to terminate. More reasonable would be for the employer requesting 90 - 120 days written notice, and for the employee to provide 90 days written notice as well.

Optimally, a contract that requires both parties to give 60 to 90 days' notice to the other party is ideal. Why? Because it will take you as a doctor at least 60 to 90 days to identify and possibly interview for a subsequent position. Whereas a 90-day notice will give you enough time to start the process of transitioning. Keep in mind that the credentialing process at your new position may take another 3 to 6 months, so you will need to plan financially if you have a break in the time between your current and next position.

When either party opts to terminate the contract, a letter of notice or notice of termination is required within a specific time frame and sent to the person specified in your contract.

Doc: Why is the termination (with or without cause) clause one of the top 5 most important terms in the contract?

Being terminated, whether it is with or without cause, is one of the most traumatizing and unexpected events for doctors to endure/manage because this is one of the few situations on the business side of medicine that we are not taught about, nor does it occur to us that we, the doctor, can actually be terminated, especially when we know and are committed to addressing the needs of our patients who need our care.

Unfortunately, life happens, which may require that you have the flexibility to terminate your contract. For example, what if I have a sick family member, get engaged, or need to move away to care for them?

Doc: Can I negotiate this termination without cause term out of my contract?

Negotiating the Termination Without Cause term out of your contract is one of the few terms that is almost always non-negotiable. Why not? Because the practice has to protect itself against adverse events, i.e., the loss of your Medicare number, termination from major insurance plans, hospital acquisitions, etc.

Therefore, it is important to be aware that you can, in fact, be terminated without cause, and your next step is to review the Term and Effects of Termination clauses within your contract in order to develop a negotiation strategy as you transition out of the practice.

So, what is important here? Let's use the RISC Analysis to find out.

o Reciprocity - The employer and the doctor-employee should be afforded the same range of days written notice to terminate the contract.
o Important - The termination clause is EXTREMELY IMPORTANT for all of the reasons cited in this section.
o Specific - The most important aspect of this clause is to know the number of days that each party must give when terminating the contract.
o Customary - Negotiating for this (or any) term to be reciprocal is standard, customary, and reasonable from a legal perspective.

TERMINATION WITH CAUSE:

Doc: *In residency, it was not a big deal if I did not complete all of my medical record charting. Now, I'm being told that my contract may not be renewed at the end of my first year in practice, mainly because I am behind on 50 charts.*

Dr. Bonnie: *(As I slap my hand to my forehead) Doc, failure to complete your medical records in a timely fashion will deeply impact your practice's ability to submit reimbursement claims in a timely fashion to ensure remittance of funds. In other words, if you don't complete your billing, the practice cannot collect the revenue that you've generated, and you become a liability. In addition, there is likely language in your contract regarding the consequences of untimely completion of medical records.*

Core Concepts: In general, most "with cause" reasons center on a doctor's:

o Noncompliance with credentialing requirements

- o Licensing matters
- o Absenteeism
- o Failure to complete medical records
- o Performance or conduct issue
- o Criminal acts
- o Impairment from drug or alcohol use, and sometimes
- o Inability to practice

Each of the "with or for cause" clauses should be written in very specific and quantifiable language.

After all, you do not want to be guilty of an infraction that you are unaware of.

There is a saying in law that applies here,
"Ignorance is not a defense."

The corollary for medicine,
"Busy is not an excuse."

We must read and remain aware of these details in order to protect our careers, our finances, and ourselves.

So, what is important here? Let's use the RISC Analysis to find out.

- o Reciprocity - The contract should contain reasons that the doctor can terminate the contract "with cause," such as breach of material (important) terms within the contract. Review this term with your health law attorney.
- o Important - The Termination With Cause clause is EXTREMELY IMPORTANT for all of the reasons cited in this section.
- o Specific - The most important aspect of this clause is to know the specific reasons for which your employment can be terminated. Be aware that certain terminations for cause get reported to the Board of Medicine and can be investigated for unprofessional conduct.

    o   Customary – Be sure to ask clarifying questions such that you fully understand the specific reasons for which you and the employer can terminate this agreement.

PROFESSIONAL LIABILITY (MALPRACTICE) INSURANCE:

Doc: I just paid $90,000 to cover my tail insurance policy after leaving my practice.

Dr. Bonnie: *Wow, Doc! My stomach is churning on your behalf.*

Core Concepts: Professional liability insurance, which is also called malpractice insurance, is one of the TOP 5 most important but least understood terms in a doctor's contract.

Malpractice Insurance <=> Liability Insurance

Some doctors choose to practice medicine without liability insurance coverage, which is called "going bare," but this can expose all of their personal property to a lawsuit.

However, the vast majority of employers, hospitals, and practices require that liability insurance policy be purchased for every doctor to protect the doctor in the event that a claim, aka lawsuit, is filed against the doctor as an individual.

In most cases for employed doctors, the practice/employer will provide professional liability insurance for its doctor-employees, given that the doctor is eligible to be underwritten for a policy. (Know what the eligibility requirements are.)

Key Components of Malpractice Insurance Policies

This section will discuss the specifics of malpractice insurance policies that are commercial policies, but not self-insured policies.

When your malpractice insurance policy is being covered (paid for) by the practice, this term in the contract should include:

- o Types of malpractice insurance policies offered will be one of the following, which will be defined in detail in the next section:
  - o An Occurrence-based insurance policy
  - o A Claims-made insurance policy
  - o An Employer-sponsored Self-Insured Malpractice insurance provided by the corporation/organization, e.g., Kaiser or other large independent health care systems
- o Limits of Liability: The limits of liability coverage will be defined by two monetary amounts, which are usually dictated by the minimum amounts required to be credentialed by the hospital/medical center where you will be working. The limits of liability will be a ratio of the amount of coverage that will be provided in a single claim and the total aggregate amount of coverage that the insurer will cover on behalf of the doctor.

For example, the limits of liability could be listed as $250,000: $750,000 or $1,000,000 : $3,000,000. Physicians in procedure-based and surgical specialties will require greater amounts of liability coverage and, therefore, will have higher limits of liability.

In addition, all entities providing medical care are required to purchase general professional liability insurance policies that insure the entire practice, including all of the doctors, nurses, medical assistants, staff, etc.

Types of Malpractice Insurance Policies Defined

An Occurrence-Based Insurance Policy

- o Covers you with liability insurance whether the claim is filed against you while you are working with the practice or whether you have transitioned to another practice. In other words, no matter when the claim occurs or is filed, an occurrence insurance policy will provide coverage to the limits of liability indicated.

○ Because this liability coverage is conferred regardless of whether you are working for the practice or if you have transitioned to another practice, a tail insurance policy is NOT required.

A Claims-Made Insurance Policy

○ Covers you with liability insurance if the claim (aka lawsuit) is filed against you while you are rendering care in a specific practice as an employee or practice owner. A claims-made policy does not cover you if any lawsuits are filed against you after you leave that place of employment. That's why you have to purchase a tail insurance policy if you have a claims-made malpractice insurance policy. It is the tail policy that covers you from any claims/lawsuits that are filed against you after you leave the practice, even if you have started working in another practice subsequently.

○ Tail coverage, which usually amounts to 2.5 times your most recent annual premium, covers both you and the practice for all occurrences and events during the duration of your employment, for a duration of two years after you leave the practice, which equals the statute of limitations for a malpractice claim.

For example, my last year of seeing patients in my orthopaedic practice, my annual premium for my annual malpractice insurance premium was $24,000. Once we decided to close the practice, I received a quote from the insurance company informing me that the cost to purchase my specific tail insurance policy would be $60,000, approximately two and a half times the amount of my annual premium. My tail coverage, which I needed to purchase to cover me for any lawsuits that were filed against me after we left the practice increased to

○ The interesting part about tail coverage is that the insurance companies usually want tail coverage to be paid for in full within 90 days of you leaving that practice.

○ There are exceptions to having to pay the full tail insurance policy. If the doctor:

- o chooses to retire from the practice of medicine (as I did), or if he or she
- o moves to a different practice where the liability insurance carrier remains the same, i.e., there is no discontinuation of liability insurance coverage necessitating a tail policy

IMPORTANT: Because tail policy coverage is so expensive, be sure that the party responsible for paying for this tail coverage is written in your contract. Ensure that this detail is in writing in your final contract before signing.

Should you leave the practice, either you as the employee or the employer will need to pay for the cost of this tail insurance. Negotiate this!

- o Ideally, the employer will agree to pay for your tail insurance at the time of your contract's expiration or non-renewal. In addition, if the employer terminates the contract without cause, it is reasonable for the employer to pay for your tail coverage. Alternatively, the employer may negotiate that if the doctor terminates the contract or resigns, then the doctor will be responsible for paying their own tail insurance.
- o Ideally, the employer will pay for it whether they terminate you or whether the contract expires, but many times a point of negotiation can be if I, as the doctor, decide to terminate this contract, I agree to pay my own malpractice. Again, I might not agree to that, especially if you're in a highly sub-specialized specialty, where your annual premiums are going to be exponentially higher, which means your tail insurance policy is going to be exorbitant. Make sure that you understand. Read through your contract. Find the type of malpractice insurance you have.

Types of Malpractice (Liability) Insurance Policies	Claims-Made	Occurrence	Self-Insured
Definition	Liability coverage is provided if the claim is made or filed while the doctor is working for the practice	Liability coverage is provided regardless of when the claim is filed or whether the doctor is employed by the employer	Liability coverage is provided regardless of when the claim is filed or whether the doctor is employed by the employer
Tail Policy Required	Yes	No	No

Figure 11 – Malpractice Insurance Comparison Table

Other Malpractice Insurance Considerations for Independent Contractors:

o If you're an independent contractor, you may be required to find, secure, and pay for your own malpractice insurance policy.

So, what is important? Let's use the RISC Analysis to find out.

o Reciprocity – Because having malpractice insurance is in the best interest of both the Employer and the Employee, malpractice provisions are usually sufficient to protect both parties. The only point of negotiation is usually the tail policy, if applicable.

o Important – If you have a claims-made policy, be sure to negotiate who will be responsible for paying for the tail insurance policy once you are no longer employed. One point of negotiation regarding malpractice insurance includes negotiating for the employer to pay for the tail insurance policy if you are terminated without cause. Work with your health lawyer to formulate your negotiation strategy.

- o Specific – These specific details about the liability insurance policy should be reflected in the agreement:
  - o The party responsible for providing malpractice insurance – the employer vs. the employee
  - o The type of malpractice insurance being offered
    - Though "self-insured" policies may or may not be spelled out in the contract, your lawyer can help you decipher whether this is a self-insurance malpractice coverage is being offered. This is important because self-insurance policies from employers operate differently than commercial insurance coverage.
  - o The limits of liability per claim and the aggregated amount
  - o Who is responsible for payment of the tail insurance policy should be clearly stated if a claims-made policy is being purchased?
  - o Customary – This is standard information that should be present in every contract. In most states, having malpractice insurance coverage is mandatory unless you live in a state where "going bare," i.e., without malpractice insurance, is allowed.

EFFECTS OF TERMINATION

Doc: *Dr. Bonnie, I couldn't take it anymore, so I just quit my job this morning!*

Dr. Bonnie: *(Slapping my hand to my forehead)...Doc, please send me your contract ASAP. This is not McDonald's. You can't JUST quit, because there are consequences written into your contract that go into effect as soon as the contract is terminated.*

Later that evening...Doc, I've read your letter of resignation that gives the practice sixty days notice; however, your contract also states that the practice can exercise the right to ask you to leave within ten days of receipt of your letter of resignation. In addition, the practice has contractually agreed to pay 25% of your tail insurance policy. Doc, are you prepared to pay the balance of your tail insurance policy?

Doc: *I don't even know what a tail policy is, much less how much it is going to cost. I also can't afford to leave this job in the next ten days.*

Dr. Bonnie: *Well, we've got a lot of strategizing to do now about your tail insurance. The good news is that once you resign with the required notice, let's say sixty days, the practice can ask you to leave before sixty days. However, they still have to pay you for the sixty days.*

I can't tell you how many of these calls I have received over the years, which is why I built an entire online course called, "Before You Resign!" I recognize that situations arise that make continued employment untenable; however, just as we have discussed throughout this book, we must be strategic if we are considering resigning or if we are notified that we are being terminated.

Either way, we have to be informed about the cascade of events that will go into place once your contract is terminated.

Conversely, when we as doctors are terminated, with or without cause, it's always a shock, and one we are generally unprepared for, because who would've thought that we would ever be fired?

Either way, some of the consequences of termination can be found in the contract term called: Effects of Termination. This is yet another critical clause that is tied to the termination clause in your contract.

Term --> Termination With and Without Cause --> Effects of Termination

I instantly review these three terms in this order when a doctor tells me that "I just quit my job," because nine times out of ten (most likely), the doctor has not reviewed their contract prior to resigning.

> Red Flag: There are other sections that require examination upon resignation, too, like restrictive covenants, non-competes, paybacks, etc., which is why it's hard to tell on your own what will happen without having our health lawyer. Remember this combination of clauses for future reference:

Core Concepts: The Effects of Termination clauses vary from contract to contract and from practice to practice. Upon termination of employment, there are three main goals that are critical for every doctor to achieve, and these include preservation and protection of our:

o Career and our future ability to become credentialed by future practices
o Medical license from a professional perspective
o Finances

Professionally, doctors have to be cautious at the point of termination because of the following possible sequelae:

o Claims of patient abandonment being levied against the doctor
o Disparaging reports being placed on the doctor's employment or credentialing files within the hospital or medical center
   o Disparaging reports being filed with the state licensing board
   o Independent contractors may not be afforded due process because they are not technically "employees"
   o Other actions that the practice may choose to exercise, if you terminate the contract

All of the above can have a powerful impact on your career and your ability to practice medicine in the future. Why? Because every credentialing committee at every future hospital or medical center is going to verify your status with each of your previous positions.

Financially, the termination of one's contract also comes with a litany of potential financial implications. One of the primary financial consequences that doctors must consider is the requisite payment of one's tail insurance policy, if the doctor has a claims-made liability insurance policy in place. Additional financial consequences of termination include:

- o The possibility of repayment of signing or relocation "bonuses" that are tied to the length of employment, which means that these are loans and not true bonuses
- o Employer's cost of replacing you and lost patient revenue without you
- o Possible payment for outstanding overhead or productivity charges from the practice, which is rare but possible

For a full list of financial considerations at the time of termination, I have created a Transition Tracker, found in Section 3 of your Power Moves Personal Workbook, which outlines 14 financial line items that doctors need to consider before resigning. It is critical that you meet with your financial advisor to construct a proforma, a projected budget, to help you and your family plan your transition strategically.

Just as we negotiated our way into our employed position, you can certainly negotiate when you need to transition out of a position. This works optimally via person-to-person engagement, which is super scary but winds up working out for the best in most situations. Resigning via email or text is not only unprofessional but may likely incite negative repercussions on behalf of the employer.

Who's Terminating the Agreement? You or the Employer?

If YOU are terminating your employment:

Before any doctor resigns from his or her position, I recommend reviewing our "Before You Resign" online course in order to build the strategy that allows you to successfully negotiate your way out of the practice with minimal professional and financial consequences.

> *Power Move #33 - If you are resigning, i.e., terminating your contract, I HIGHLY recommend that you resign in person FIRST, then submit a written letter of resignation NEXT. This direct person to person approach, followed by written documentation, will hopefully help to mitigate any potential negative consequences of your resignation.*

If the EMPLOYER is terminating your employment:

First, review the critical clauses that will inform you of your rights upon termination:

Term --> Termination With and Without Cause --> Effects of Termination

Make sure that you respond to the termination notice, ideally in person, then in writing, so that you can negotiate your transition where possible to do so.

> *Power Move #34 - If the employer is terminating you without cause, then a point of negotiation before you even sign the initial contract is to assert that if the employer terminates your contract,*
> *then the employer:*
> *Nullifies the non-compete clause*
> *Covers the cost of your tail policy, if applicable.*

So what is important here? Let's use the RISC Analysis to find out:

o Reciprocity - Be sure to understand what the employer asserts as its rights upon termination of your employment.

For Educational Purposes Only. Not Intended as Legal Advice.

> Conversely, understand what your rights are upon termination, as well.

- o Important – Regardless of whether you or your employer terminates your employment/contract, be sure to NEGOTIATE the terms of the termination, as described above.
- o Specific – Specific details regarding the consequences of termination should be clear to you upon reviewing your contract.
- o Customary – This is standard information that should be present in every contract, please look for it and make sure that you know what your rights are.

RESTRICTIVE COVENANTS

Next, we will discuss three of the most common terms that literally restrict the doctor's actions once a contract is terminated. These restrictive covenants, especially the covenant not-to-compete, definitely meet the criteria for one of the Top 5 most important contract terms that every doctor must know.

COVENANT NOT-TO-COMPETE = NON-COMPETE CLAUSE

The covenant not to compete, aka the non-compete clause, is one of many terms that fall under the umbrella of restrictive covenants found in doctor employment agreements.

In an attempt to protect their market share of patients within a given region and for a given time frame, employers will incorporate a non-compete clause into the employed doctor's contract. This clause states that you will not practice within a certain mile radius that's called the geographic scope, for a certain period of time, called the duration, within proximity of that hospital system or practice site.

Why? Consider this scenario – In addition to protecting their patient base, employers also want to protect their investment. Hospitals and other employers incur transition costs to the tune of six to seven figures when bringing a doctor on board as an employee. The employer certainly would not want you to leave their organization having been trained with their insights, just for you to go and join a competing organization, after all of the resources and investment that they put into you.

Covenants not-to-compete should be reviewed for the following:

- o Radius of prohibition
  - o Geographical – based on miles or the specific exclusion of certain counties
  - o Competitors – specifying a particular competing hospital or medical entity (and their affiliates) for which a doctor could not work after leaving a practice
- o Duration of prohibition – specified as the number of years during which the doctor cannot compete with the organization
- o Delineation of Excluded Medical Services – specifies the types of medical services that a doctor cannot provide after leaving the practice within the radius and duration of prohibition defined in this covenant.

Exercise/Homework: Before signing any contract, take time to draw the specified radius around the practice location (and its satellites or affiliated locations on a map, so that you can understand the scope of the geographic non-compete. This can also be accomplished via Google).

Primary Practice (Site) Designation: This is another important stipulation for your covenant not-to-compete is that you want to have added on to that part of the agreement. This designation says that when your employment term ends that you agree not to practice within a certain number of miles of the PRIMARY location where you see patients.

Many of these hospital systems and group practices have satellites throughout the states now. If you draw a 10-mile radius around each and every one of those practice locations, that means you'll be driven very likely out of that state and sometimes out of the entire region. You want to be aware of that and request that the non-compete only applies to where you see the majority of your patients most of the time. That's called a primary site designation. Additionally, the duration says for two years. You'll want to talk to your Health Law attorney to find out if that's customary.

The non-compete essentially indicates that the doctor cannot provide any medical services of any kind for any entity that offers healthcare during that period of time within that radius. This is comprehensively restrictive and can really be prohibitive in allowing the doctor to live and work comfortably within a desired location.

> Red Flag: If you see a restrictive covenant like this, that's also a Red Flag. If a practice is being that prohibitive, it's just not reasonable to be restricted to render healthcare.

But if, let's say, you're a cardiologist, you could say, "I agree not to offer cardiology services within that 10-mile radius for 24 months." But maybe you can work in an emergency room or an urgent care center, where you're not practicing specifically cardiology, but that might be a way for you to carve out the opportunity to still practice if you absolutely need to stay in that area.

> *Power Move #35* - *While non-competes are usually not negotiated out of doctor employment contracts, the radius, duration, and medical services prohibited can usually be negotiated into terms that are agreeable to both parties by providing valid professional and/or personal reasons.*

For example, if a doctor is looking forward to joining a practice in the DC area so that she can be close to family, then it is reasonable to negotiate a significantly smaller radius of prohibition such that the doctor could remain in the DC region, i.e., in Maryland or Virginia to practice, should this position not work out.

Can I negotiate the non-compete clause out of my contract?

Not likely. "I don't want a restrictive covenant at all." Out of the ... I can't even tell you how many contracts I have reviewed over time, well over 100 contracts, I've only seen one where there was no restrictive covenant.

You're usually not going to be able to get that negotiated out, unless you're also in one of those states where non-competes cannot be upheld. States where non-competes are not enforceable include California, North Dakota and Oklahoma. States where limited circumstances govern the enforceability of non-compete clauses include:

- o   Non-compete clauses disallowed for all employees (e.g. California, Oklahoma, North Dakota)
- o   Non-compete clauses disallowed for physicians (e.g. Massachusetts, Delaware, Colorado, Rhode Island)
- o   Physician non-compete clauses are permitted, but subject to stricter standards than general employees e.g. Tennessee, Texas, New Mexico and Connecticut[6]

Exceptions where the non-compete clause may not be enforced include situations where the doctor leaves the practice and either:

- o   Accepts a position at a Veterans Hospital or other government facility
- o   University position
- o   Starts their own practice or joins a small private practice

What happens if the non-compete is violated?

The employer can sue the doctor and their new employer for breach of contract, alleging monetary damages against both parties. Alternatively, the new employer and doctor can agree to buy out the doctor from their current practice to avoid being sued for damages. However, some contracts have steep liquidated damages penalties that can be up to your last year's salary too.

These clauses are totally legal and are NOT routinely thrown out of court when contested. They protect the practice from undue competition should you leave the practice. Note that there is ALWAYS a penalty in place for breaking a non-compete, so understand the terms. Also, keep in mind that fighting a non-compete contractual clause takes time and money with no guarantee of success. Be aware also that courts consider the employer to have a genuine business interest in protecting their business with non-competes.

I will end this section on an interesting side note by letting doctors know that non-compete clauses are not customary or standard in the legal field, i.e., attorneys do not sign, nor do they agree to having non-compete clauses in their contracts. Go figure!

So, what is important here? Let's use the RISC Analysis to find out:

- o Reciprocity – Be sure to understand what the employer asserts as its rights upon termination of your employment. Conversely, understand what your rights are upon termination, as well.
- o Important – The key components of a sample non-compete:
  - o Radius of prohibition = 150 miles
  - o Duration of prohibition = 2 years
  - o Delineation of Excluded Medical Services = all medical services
- o Specific – Consider negotiating in a primary practice site designation provision, as described above, into the non-compete clause of your contract
- o Customary – Non-compete clauses, aka non-competition covenants, restrictive covenants, are customary and standard, except in the states where they are not lawfully upheld (or are upheld in limited circumstances), which are California, Oklahoma, North Dakota, and Montana[7].

NON-DISCLOSURE AND NON-SOLICITATION:

Practices and their attorneys take measures to protect their business systems/operations, patient information, intellectual property, patients, and employees, all of which are deemed as "assets" to the practice. The courts consider these reasonable business interests that employers are entitled to protect. These restrictive covenants limit the actions of the doctor-employee with respect to these "assets."

The non-disclosure term does the following:

o Identifies penalties for disseminating the practice's proprietary information, trade secrets, intellectual or physical property after leaving the practice.
o Prohibits the discussion of any information pertaining to the business or operations of the practice, usually for a period of 2 years after termination.
o This provision or in a separate term will also address the handling or mishandling of Protected Health Information (PHI).

Important: The non-disclosure term is NOT the same as the Health Insurance Portability and Accountability Act (HIPAA), which are federally mandated regulations conferring privacy and protection for patient's health information.

The non-solicitation term does the following:

o Prohibits an employee from hiring or engaging in business arrangements with other employees of the practice once a doctor leaves the practice or from soliciting patients to leave with the leaving doctor for a specified period of time.

So, what is important here? Let's use the RISC Analysis to find out.

o Reciprocity – Opportunities for reciprocity are fairly limited when it comes to restrictive covenants, such as non-disclosure and non-solicitation.
o Important – Of course, it is important to understand the terms, such as these restrictive covenants, which govern the doctor's actions upon leaving employment by imposing consequences, so we need to know that they are.

o Specific – As in the non-compete clause, be sure to review the duration of the prohibited actions regarding area and type of work: restricted, non-disclosure, confidentiality, and non-solicitation.

o Customary – Yes, these covenants are customary, but your attorney will review the extent of the restrictions to determine the legality of the restrictions under federal and state laws.

EMPLOYMENT

Doc: When I signed the contract, I had no idea that I was being employed as an independent contractor. I thought all employment was the same. Now I have a $75,000 tax bill. What did I miss in my contract?

Dr. Bonnie: This is one of those situations where we don't know what we don't know. As a result, many doctors have experienced negative tax and other financial consequences due to not understanding the nuances of their employment.

Core Concepts: Please take the time to review your agreement for the type of employment in which you are engaging in with the other party identified in the first paragraph of the agreement.

> *Power Move #36 - Be aware that all contract language is not this clear. Take the time to clarify whether you are an employee or an independent contractor for yourself.*

Employment vs. Independent Contractor – Please review Chapter 5 for the critical details that differentiate these two types of employment.

In addition, here are some key questions, which should be asked based on the type of practice that you seek to join:

o Will you be an employee vs. an independent contractor?

o   If you are transitioning into private practice, is partnership an option? If so, when and how is partnership determined?
o   Especially if you are going into academics, what title will you hold in this position (which is always negotiable, btw)?
o   If you are moving into a leadership position, what will your title(s) be and in association with which institutions, medical schools, or hospitals?

So, what is important? Let's use the RISC Analysis to find out.

o   Reciprocity – This term of the contract should specify the employer's obligations regarding tax withholdings and other deductions for benefits for employed physicians. Alternatively, for independent contractors, the correlating term may or may not describe each party's responsibilities with regards to tax withholdings and other deductions for benefits if you are an independent contractor.
o   Important – Identification of the employment type is critical because if you are an independent contractor, your taxes, benefits, and malpractice insurance coverage are not the responsibility of the employer.
o   Specific – Thus, I recommend working with an accountant before you sign the contract to determine the amount and frequency of your tax payments, and you will need to secure your own health insurance and retirement vehicles.
o   Customary – This is standard information that should be present in every contract, please look for it and make sure that you know what you are signing up for.

DUTIES AND RESPONSIBILITIES:

Doc: Under this section of my contract, it only indicates that I will render medical services. Isn't this sufficient since I am an internal medicine physician?

Dr. Bonnie: The reference to medical services is so vague and can be defined widely, so you should request a more detailed and definitive description of your duties and responsibilities. Though you are an internist, the scope of medical services could extend from primary care to specialty or surgical services. Please clarify all duties and responsibilities with the potential employer.

Core Concepts: This term describes the occupational duties and responsibilities that are a regular part of one's employment.

The doctor's duties and responsibilities as an employee should be detailed and include specifics, such as:

- o The scope of your clinical, teaching, administrative responsibilities to the practice, i.e., productivity benchmarks, teaching hours, supervisory of mid-levels, administrative/meeting requirements should be outlined here in detail.
- o Your percentage of full-time equivalent (FTE) or specific work hours
- o Your doctor and/or administrative supervisor/manager whom you will report to should be listed here as well.
- o If you will have responsibilities in more than one location, this is where the locations and requisite responsibilities should be identified.
- o Any on-call duties should also be indicated.

These are the types of nebulous phrases that can end up causing doctors significant distress if we are suddenly assigned to work at a location or multiple locations that we weren't anticipating having to commute to or from, which thereby limits or affects our personal time. Then, the spiral begins.

Let's avoid the spiral and ask all of these clarifying questions BEFORE we sign any agreement.

So, what is important here? Let's use the RISC Analysis to find out. Reciprocally, this section will outline the practice's responsibilities to you:

- o Administrative and or clinical support, administrative medical assistant support
- o Training and onboarding support

- o Oversight of mid-levels
- o Computer or other digital supplies
- o Productivity reporting
- o Performance evaluation criteria and timing of reviews
- o Important – Based on the details listed in this term, the doctor-employee should be crystal clear about what the potential employer's expectations are of the doctor. Key terms from the Duties and Responsibilities term of your contract should include:
  - o Benchmarks- another word for baselines used for comparison
  - o FTE – Full-time equivalent
  - o Your supervisor, i.e., reporting responsibilities
  - o Definition of on-call duties
- o Specific – Specific clinical, teaching, and administrative duties should be listed here in no uncertain terms. When and where you are to fulfill these duties should also be defined.
- o Customary – This is standard information that should be present in every contract, please look for it and make sure that you know what you are signing up for. Not being clear on your duties and responsibilities is a huge course of discouragement for doctors, because if you are unclear about your duties or if the duties continually change, this creates stress and undoubtedly affects our health, personal time, and lives.

OWNERSHIP OPPORTUNITY:

Private practices, ranging from 1 to over 100 doctors, may offer an opportunity for a new doctor to become a partner, think "partial owner" of the practice and its assets.

The following terms may be used interchangeably:

- o Partner
- o Owner
- o Shareholder

The process of becoming a partner, owner, or shareholder is different for every practice. However, the generally accepted process usually takes place in two steps:

1. The doctor initially becomes an employee of the practice.
   a. Essentially this is the trial period where you, the doctor, observe the practice and its operations to determine whether you want to become a partner or owner in this practice. The practice is assessing you as to whether you are a good fit for the practice as well.
   b. Also, during this initial employment period, the doctor is working to satisfy the partnership eligibility requirements, which should be clearly outlined in the employment agreement.
2. Once the eligibility requirements are met, the doctor is eligible to become a partner, and the practice proceeds with the steps to conferring partnership status to the doctor.

The opportunity to become a partial owner should be outlined in the employment agreement, and may detail one or more of these examples of eligibility requirements (which vary highly from practice to practice) in order to become a partner:

○ The number of years a doctor must work and the productivity benchmarks that must be achieved in order to be eligible for partnership
○ The equity arrangement
○ If the route to partnership requires a buy-inn (payment from the potential partner to purchase equity in the practice's assets), the following should be specified in the contract:
  ○ buy-in contingencies at the end of your employment term
  ○ how the buy-in will be calculated
    ▪ If a specific dollar amount is indicated, this is a RED FLAG!!!! Changing practice dynamics over time makes it impossible for any practice to estimate a buy-in amount at some time in the future. As stated above, a buy-in

> calculation should be indicated instead of a
> specific dollar amount.
> o The time frame of the practice's offer and the transfer
> of ownership

So, what is important here? Let's use the RISC Analysis to find out.

- o Reciprocity – The ownership opportunity, i.e., the details on how you can become a partial owner in the practice or entity, should be described in the initial employment contract. However, once you satisfy the eligibility requirements to become a partner, you will likely sign a second, separate partnership agreement that will outline the practice's obligations to you as a partner and reciprocally, your obligations to the practice as a partner.
- o Important – For those who are interested, the road to becoming a partner, owner, or shareholder in a practice should be clearly outlined from the start of your contractual relationship with a practice.
- o Specific – Unclear or non-specific eligibility requirements, poor or nebulous descriptions of the practice's assets, including goodwill buy-ins, non-quantifiable assets, should be clarified and viewed as Red Flags.
- o Customary – If applicable, it is recommended that the method of calculating the amount of a doctor's buy-in into a practice be outlined during one's initial negotiations with a practice.

INTELLECTUAL PROPERTY:

Doc: I just launched my dream invention, which is going to be sold online, but I forgot to check the intellectual property clause in my contract. Can I negotiate to have my IP carved out of my contract after I have signed my contract?

Dr. Bonnie: Yes, I would encourage everyone to always renegotiate his or her contract, most effectively done during your annual renewal period, which will cost you the expense of re-engaging your health law attorney (highly recommended). However, it is best to negotiate for ownership of your own IP before you sign your initial contract, when you have the most leverage.

Intellectual property includes copyrights, trademarks, inventions, or other proprietary products that could possibly be licensed or monetized in the future.

As aspiring doctors, we have always been intellectually and creatively curious leaders and problem-solvers, drivers of solutions and innovators with multiple intelligences that we should continue exercising even after we become an employed doctor. We should be able to retain the rights to our intellectual property from our brain power. The fact that we are working for an employer doesn't give the employer the right to own that UNLESS you have created your IP from patients' data, operations, or anything that could be shown to have contributed to the development of the IP. You do have a right to own what you create on your own time, with none of their resources or information.

Traditionally, academic institutions rightfully assert ownership of the intellectual property created if one invents or develops a new innovation while working within their resourceful academic environment. Many 21st-century doctor employers, not just those in academic centers, are now claiming ownership of a doctor's intellectual property, regardless of whether it is medically or clinically related to their work or not. I have seen practices assert ownership of the intellectual property of doctors, not only if they are full-time employees, but that of part-time employees and independent contractors.

> *Power Move #37 - If you have any current or potential projects in development that are eligible to be patented, trademarked, for copyright with the potential for monetization, please develop your own list of intellectual property and proprietary works for submission as a "carve out."*

I would like to encourage all of you, doctors, to protect your intellectual property, or there should be some means for you to at least negotiate that point with your potential employer. Again, it is not as easy with academic institutions, but I have seen some academic institutions now ease up on the absolute requirement that all IP belongs to the organization or academic institution. So, be ready to negotiate after building a negotiating strategy with your health law attorney.

See the Power Moves Intellectual Property "Carve Out" List in Appendix I for examples of potential proprietary works to be listed in a contractual carve-out appendix or addendum that a doctor could develop and subsequently copyright, trademark, or patent.

OUTSIDE REVENUE GENERATION

Related to intellectual property ownership, doctors should scour their contracts for the terms that regulate our ability to generate outside revenue via additional revenue sources such as:

- o Employment opportunities, e.g., working as an independent contractor in an outpatient or urgent care center
- o Speaking engagements
- o Primary or Affiliate Product Sales
- o Consulting

So, what is important here? Let's use the RISC Analysis to find out.

- o Reciprocity – Proactively plan to negotiate for your right to own your intellectual property, just as employers have been increasingly asserting their rights to do so.
- o Important – This is one of the key terms of the contract that confers protection to the doctor. Be sure to negotiate for your right to own your current and future intellectual property, independent of your employer.
- o Specific – Create a detailed list of the potential IP that you are or have dreamed about developing or creating. Keep a

running log of these ideas so that it is easily accessible when it is time to negotiate or renegotiate your contract.

o Customary – Just to reiterate, it has now become customary for employers of all types to assume ownership of the doctor-employee's intellectual property. Be sure to review this term and negotiate for the right to retain ownership of your own brainpower.

ADDITIONAL CONTRACT TERMINOLOGY TO BE REVIEWED BY YOU AND YOUR HEALTH LAW ATTORNEY

Having reviewed the critical terms within an employment contract that ALL doctors should review, prior to meeting with their health law attorney, here is a list of additional contract terms that are likely to appear in your employment contract. While every term in a contract is important, the following are terms that are more or less standard contract language, i.e., legalese that your attorney can review with you with relative efficiency during one of your contract consultations.

o Assignability
o Representations of Physician
o Medical Records
o Equipment – office, computers, phone
o Notices
o Severability
o Waiver
o Governing Law; Jurisdiction; Venue

SIGNATURES

At the end of the body of the contract and before the appendices/addenda is the page for the signatures from representatives from both of the parties defined in the very first paragraph of the contract.

Contracts are not executed (valid or enforceable) until BOTH parties have signed the contract or agreement.

> ***Power Move for Independent Contractors #38*** - *The signatures, titles, and dates of the signatures are required from both parties. Please note, if you are signing an agreement as an independent contractor who has his or her own corporate entity, such as an LLC, you should sign as a representative of your company, and not as an individual. Please work with your accountant to determine which corporate entity is best for you BEFORE signing any document.*

Though it sounds silly, many of us fail to obtain an executed copy of the contract because the negotiation process may have been protracted or, more commonly, we just get busy. However, it is critical to obtain a valid copy of the executed contract, so that you will have the final version that was agreed upon in case you need to refer back to the contract in the future.

Don't forget to initial every page of the contract upon signing to make sure that pages are not added or deleted when final signatures are being obtained. #doctorprotectthyself

Finally, in Appendix A, I thought that it would be important to provide an abbreviated but realistic example of a contract incorporating the contract terms that will be defined throughout the chapter. Please refer back to this sample contract as a reference when reviewing each contract term being discussed. I have also included a Terminology Checklist in Workbook 2 to serve as an outline for you to complete while analyzing each term of this sample employment contract.

CHAPTER SUMMARY

POWER MOVES

o Every doctor is capable of developing a baseline understanding of the above 18 contract terms. Hopefully, this chapter has helped to propel you toward this end.

TAKE-HOME POINTS

o After reviewing your contract using this chapter as your primary resource, you can now have an informed conversation with your health law attorney to make sure that your needs and wants have been integrated within the contract.

RED FLAGS

o Review these 18 terms for their respective Red Flags that you should discuss specifically with your health law attorney.

HOMEWORK

o With your new foundation of knowledge and playbook of power moves, your next step will be to have a series of critical conversations during the negotiation process of finding your first position. Section 3 of this book will go into detail on how to formulate a winning negotiation strategy

REFERENCES

6. Habig, A. https://freedomhealthworks.com/2020/01/07/the-curtail-abuse-of-physician-non-compete-agreements/
7. https://www.beckreedriden.com/wp-content/uploads/2019/04/Noncompetes-50-State-Survey-Chart-20190427.pdf

NOTES

_____

_____

_____

_____

_____

_____

_____

_____

_____

_____

_____

_____

_____

_____

_____

_____

_____

_____

_____

_____

_____

_____

_____

Chapter 9

COMPENSATION MODELS

Doc: *With all of this delayed gratification and student loan debt, I am ready to just sign my contract and GET PAID!!!*

Dr. Bonnie: *Got it! However, I want you to understand that HOW you will get paid can be complex and that your salary is not always guaranteed. It can actually be quite complicated. Lets explore.*

This chapter is for our new doctors, or doctors early in their career, who are moving into a six-figure salary compensation for the first time after completing their training. This is also for doctors who may be transitioning from one type of practice to another to ensure you are clear about what to expect.

In today's healthcare environment, compensation for physicians has become a complex subject. The goal of this chapter is to help doctors understand the following aspects of how we are compensated, including:

- o How to calculate the total value of a compensation package
- o What relevant questions should be asked to help determine compensation amounts
- o How to understand the current models used to derive compensation models

PART 1 – UNDERSTANDING COMPENSATION

As we alluded to earlier, we are comparing our compensation to the body's extremities, the parts that drive motion and propel us forward. Certainly, we can view compensation as the fuel that powers the work we do in service to our patients.

Compensation provides us with stability in our careers, finances, retirement, health, well-being, continuing education, etc. One can clearly see that many aspects of life are affected by how we negotiate our compensation package; it's not just about the salary.

The Total Compensation Package

Thus, when an offer is received, our goal is to calculate the total value of the entire compensation package that you are being offered. The total value of the compensation package includes the totality of the quantifiable components that represent income to the doctor. (See Figure 12 and Appendix H)

Components of a Compensation Package Blueprint

Total Compensation Package Value = Salary + Benefits + Leave + Miscellaneous

Components of a Compensation Package

Salary	Benefits (Cont.)
• Base Pay	• Retirement Contributions
○ Salary vs. Income Guarentee	○ +/- matching funds
○ Gross vs. Net	○ 401k , 403b, Pension
• Variable Pay	
○ Signing Bonus	**Leave**
○ Productivity Bonus	
○ Loan Repayment	○ Admin CME -- +/- pd fees
Benefits	○ Sick, Family Maternity Personal
• Insurance	○ Dues, Licenses
○ Malpractice	○ Moving Expenses
○ Life, Disability, Health, Unemployment, Worker's Compensation	○ Cell phone, parking, meals, travel, (airfare, company car)

Figure 12: Components of a Compensation Package Blueprint

The components of your compensation package can be reviewed in 4 subsets of the compensation package, including:

- Salary
- Benefits
- Leave
- Miscellaneous

Notice that the salary is but one component of the compensation package. The good news is that your team of trusted advisors can provide the monetary values of the numerous components in the compensation package, thereby allowing you to have greater leverage when comparing one contract to another during your negotiations.

> **Power Move #39** - *Calculate the total value of your compensation package, which is not just the salary amount in your paycheck.*

Each component of your compensation package can be assigned a dollar figure, and this is where we should work with our financial advisors and accountants to quantify the annual monetary value of the retirement and health benefits being offered.

It is also extremely important to work with a tax accountant, who is abreast of the most current tax laws and changes, to quantify in dollars and cents the tax liability that we will incur if we accept either a signing or relocation bonuses (aka loans in some cases), loan repayment or loan forgiveness.

Why? Because ALL compensation, including loan principles and interest in repayment or forgiveness, is taxable. For additional understanding of this particular point, please read and discuss this online article by Stephanie M. Sharp, "The Forgivable Loan: A Recruitment Tool with Tax Implications For Physicians And Employers."

> **Power Move #40** - *Be sure to review each aspect of your compensation with your accountant, financial advisor, and attorney in order to understand the tax implications, budgetary impacts, and legalities of your compensation package.*

Now that we have insight into all of the components of your compensation package, please review the Power Moves Needs and Wants Blueprint (yes, that again) to help identify which components of the compensation package are of most importance in order to customize our negotiations to meet your needs.

Taking the above steps to being strategic and proactive into account when considering a compensation package, versus simply reacting to a compensation offer that is presented to you.

Our Worth

Doc: How do I know what the fair market value for my salary is?

Dr. Bonnie: By doing your due diligence, i.e., research, and through comparing multiple employment offers, we can collect our own data, which will provide us with a sound basis for our negotiation.

Physicians are the primary revenue generators in the US healthcare system. In fact, according to a 2019 Physician Inpatient/Outpatient Revenue Study by Merrit Hawkins,

"The average (revenue generation) for all types of doctors tracked in the survey is $2,378,727 per year. This includes both net inpatient and outpatient revenue derived from hospital admissions, tests, treatments, prescriptions, and procedures performed or ordered by doctors."

Ref: *https://www.merritthawkins.com/news-and-insights/thought-leadership/survey/2019-doctor-inpatient-outpatient-revenue-survey/*

From family medicine to cardiovascular surgeons, doctors generate 5 – 10 times our annual salaries for the hospital, university, or others per this report, and this is where our monetary value lies within the healthcare paradigm.

Thus, it is important for us to negotiate for compensation that is in alignment with the fair market value (i.e., the customary salary range for doctors in our specialty in the same type of practice and practice location or site), in lieu of settling for the first salary that is offered.

Hospitals and medical centers, especially those that are non-profit organizations, are regulated by law with regard to how fair market value is determined and what amount of compensation that can be offered. Be aware that physician compensation can be different within the same facility for the same services based on a number of factors.

More specifically, the following are the most common sources referred to in order to find standard doctor compensation data:

o American Association of Medical Colleges compensation data for academic doctors, which is available to faculty leadership, including Chairs and Designated Institutional Officers

o Specialty Associations – National specialty associations customarily collect data regarding their doctor's compensation, practice types and other practice details

o Local Medical Associations – Many Chief Medical Officers and doctor liaisons (i.e., recruiters) belong to local medical associations; thus, the associations may have access to local doctor compensation data

o Merritt Hawkins – Research and publish annual doctor compensation surveys based on data received from doctors and healthcare administrators

o Medscape – Online Physician Surveys, which are usually specialty-specific

o Physician Colleagues – Physicians who have recently transitioned into the workforce are bountiful sources of information, especially those who are in your same specialty and who work in a similar type of practice. Having most recently interviewed at a number of practices, inquiring with your network of doctor-colleagues could prove to be a huge resource.

For those considering offers from hospitals or medical centers, here are other key questions you should ask:

o How does the hospital determine the fair market value of compensation?

o What is the average annual compensation of doctors in their second or third year of practice? Do they meet their productivity minimums?

IMPORTANT: When it comes to determining the amount of compensation offered to a physician, employers cannot exceed the Fair Market Value compensation to any physician, hence the first question above. In addition, when hiring/employing physicians, employers must not violate:

- o Federal Stark Laws
- o Anti-kickback Statutes
- o IRS private benefit guidance, for non-profit organizations

These further underscores the importance of having a health law attorney review our employment agreement to ensure that the employer is in compliance with all of the above, otherwise our individual medical license and career could be in jeopardy.

For those considering offers from private practices, where partnership is an option, here are additional questions that should be asked:
- o How long does it take to gain partnership?
- o What is the total compensation expected each year until partnership (i.e., understanding levels of incentive compensation and the likelihood of payment)? After partnership?
- o What are the criteria for becoming a partner?
- o Is there a buy-in required to become a partner? How is the buy-in calculated?

Components of a Compensation Package

SALARY - *Show me the money!!!*

Total compensation is equal to the total compensation package that we have been discussing.

Components of your salary will include:

- o Fixed (Base) salary – the amount paid at fixed intervals
  - o Gross salary – the pre-tax amount offered in your contract

o Net salary – your take-home salary after Federal taxes, State taxes, and deductions have been withheld and paid by the employer
o Variable pay
    o Signing bonus
    o Productivity bonus
    o Loan Repayment options
    o On-call Duties

Fixed Salary, aka Base Salary

One's salary is defined as a fixed periodical compensation to be paid for services rendered and is but one component of the total compensation.

The base pay being offered is a gross salary amount that does NOT take into account your tax liabilities and other payroll deductions for health or retirement benefits. It is up to you to calculate your NET take-home salary, based on the number of withholdings and the amounts for benefits that you elect to deduct. Note: this is where you make a call to your accountant to help you determine these dollar amounts.

> Red Flag: Another critical point is to determine whether this salary is guaranteed or whether this is an income guarantee, which is a compensation model used by hospital systems to entice doctors to work in rural and sometimes underserved areas. I bring this up, because income guarantees are actually loans. We will discuss this more later in this chapter.

Variable Pay

Variable pay, aka incentive pay options, are compensation components of the salary which may fluctuate and are the compensation components which can usually be negotiated:

- Signing bonus – Traditionally, signing bonuses constituted one-time bonus payments provided to the doctor upon signing of the employment contract. Increasingly, signing (and other) bonuses are being offered contingent on either:
  - time – the bonus requires that the doctor work for a practice for a specific term
  - repayment – the "bonus" is actually a LOAN that is repaid with interest on a monthly basis
- Productivity bonus – Being paid based on doctor-productivity can be a volume-based approach to compensation. Productivity bonuses can be based on:
  - actual collections of fees/revenue,
  - grant/research revenue, or
  - Relative Value Units, aka RVUs, a measure of physician's productivity.
- Productivity-based compensation and bonuses require that the doctor generate and surpass a specified number of RVUs, but each doctor has to understand:
  - How are RVUs calculated in each practice?
  - Are you compensated based on the number of RVUs that you bill for versus the amount of revenue that is collected based on the RVUs you generate?
  - How many RVUs are generated annually by current doctors in this practice who are in my same specialty?
  - Based on the minimum RVU requirement in the agreement, how many patients must be seen, and how many procedures are required to meet this RVU requirement?
- Loan Repayment options – Loan repayment and loan forgiveness options may be available from the employer. Both are considered income and are thus taxable.
- Administrative Duties – Physician leadership is critical. Inquiring about an opportunity to earn additional compensation for administrative services (i.e., medical director) is encouraged.
- On-Call Duties – Pay for overnight on-call duties is becoming more of a standard, but I would encourage

doctors to absolutely negotiate for hourly pay for time spent on-call.

o   Charitable or free care – The employer may ask you to do a certain amount of uncompensated care or surgery. Note that those associated RVUs will not be counted towards your target number of RVUs.

> **Red Flag:** More and more frequently, signing and relocation and relocation "bonuses" are being tied to requisite time commitment obligations, otherwise the bonus must be repaid. This means that this "bonus" is actually a type of forgivable loan. Loans of any type usually require specific and sometimes separate documentation within the contract, usually in the form of a promissory note.

Promissory notes are loan documents that must grab our attention, because this is the document that outlines a financial obligation that we are committing to, so we must carefully review these documents with our lawyer, financial advisor and tax accountant BEFORE ever signing a promissory note.

> **Red Flag:** Be sure to know what is the target number of RVUs you need to accrue before your compensation will be decreased or increased. Can you reach that target? If not, negotiate a reasonable

For those considering employment offers from hospitals or medical centers, here are other key questions you should ask:

o   How does the hospital determine the fair market value of compensation?

o   What is the average annual compensation of doctors after 2, 5 and 10 years?

FRINGE BENEFITS:

In reference to an employment arrangement, the term "fringe benefits" applies to the extra benefits an employee receives that is in addition to salary. The law requires that all employees in the same employment category be offered the same benefits. That doesn't mean you will get all those benefits. It will be up to you to decide if you want them and how much will be deducted from your salary to pay for those benefits you are eligible for. Employers are not required to offer any benefits, and they can change them at any time, as long as they do the same for all employees in the same category.

For doctors, benefits comprise a major subset of the total compensation and include practice/income protections and retirement provisions, such as:

- Liability insurance
- Health, dental, and vision insurance
- Life insurance
- Disability insurance
- Long term care insurance
- Retirement/Savings Plans
    - e.g. 401k, 403b or other
    - Thrift Savings Plans
- Flexible Spending Accounts
    - Healthcare or Dependent Care
- Continuing Medical Education Credits (CMEs)
- Association membership dues, subscriptions, and payments for licenses
- Paid Time Off (PTO)

For many doctors, these benefits rise to the top of our priority lists during contract negotiations for any number of reasons.

For example, shortly after I was married, my husband took a new position. Because of my rheumatoid arthritis, it was very important to us that he review the contract thoroughly and negotiate for the best health insurance plan available with his new employer. Because I had been paying for COBRA insurance and because the costs of my medications were exorbitant, having ideal health benefits were far more important than focusing primarily on salary being offered.

For doctor-employees, calculate the total compensation derived from your benefits package with the help of your financial advisor and accountant. Interestingly, a couple of doctors whom I have coached have opted for a stronger benefits package while accepting a moderate salary because of their specific needs and wants for themselves and their families. For example, maternity leave or flexible time to accommodate childcare hours.

DEFERRED COMPENSATION/RETIREMENT CONTRIBUTIONS:

Regarding retirement contributions, if you encounter an organization that is willing to match any contributions, it is highly recommended. As an aside, it is highly recommended that you maximize your contributions in which your employer will match the amount of funds that you are putting into your retirement account.

Here are some sample key questions regarding the retirement benefits offered:

- o Does the organization offer 401k, 403b, pensions, or other retirement vehicles?
- o When does the employee become vested in those retirement accounts? In other words, how long do you have to be there in order for you to essentially own the monies that you are contributing to the retirement plan from your paycheck?
- o Does the employer match contributions from the employee?

Benefits Considerations for Independent Contractors

Independent contractors customarily need to secure and pay their own benefits based on the GROSS salary that is received as compensation; therefore, it is customary for independent contractors to be paid slightly more than employees who may generally be doing the same type of work because they do not routinely receive benefits. You may still be eligible for benefits, depending on the employer. Ask for that. Sometimes there are productivity bonuses. Ask if you want them.

> Red Flag: Some contractors are paid hourly. Watch out for contracts that limit the number of hours you will be paid, but keep in mind that you still have to stay to write notes to complete your records, which may extend beyond these work hours.

> Red Flag: Many doctors, who work as independent contractors, fail to accurately calculate the amount of compensation that they will need in order to secure their own insurance protections and to pay for their own taxes on either a quarterly or annual basis.

LEAVE:

Core Concepts: Leave, also known as paid time off (PTO), is many times inclusive of educational (CME time), vacation, personal leave, which may include sick leave at some institutions. Standard leave is considered to average approximately 2 - 4 weeks annually, with 3 weeks being most common. Consider 4 weeks to be great.

- o If you are under a productivity compensation model, keep in mind that 4 weeks equals a month. The more time you take off, the harder it becomes to reach bonus levels.
- o Restrictions on the number of consecutive days off may be specified. Why? Because there will be a definite, negative effect on the cash flow of the practice if you take off too many days in a row.

Leave can be used to serve any number of purposes, including:

- o Personal leave
- o Educational leave
- o Maternity/Paternity leave

Many employers are combining personal leave to include any and all sick, family, maternity, paternity, or vacation leave. They package all of that into one set time frame for you to split up according to your own desires. Find out the standard amount of time in your particular specialty, in your particular region, or in the type of employment that you have.

Standard educational leave allows you to attend educational conferences, to obtain CME courses that you might take online, and if you negotiate it in, for the organization to offer you a certain amount of compensation to pay for these CME, either conferences or online courses.

Based on your contract and how many weeks are indicated, any additional time that you take off will not be paid time off.

RELOCATION EXPENSES:

While customary, moving expenses will include the cost of moving you to another city; however, you will likely have to negotiate for the move of your family. These expenses do NOT customarily include a separate move for a significant other from another city.

- o A specific formula should be indicated with or without a cap versus a specific dollar amount.
- o Alternatively, you should be allowed to obtain bids from 3 moving companies and choose the company you want within the average price range. This will be far more feasible for you rather than finding a moving company to move you for a specific dollar amount. This is in lieu of accepting a specific dollar amount. By obtaining three estimates, you will obtain an approximate cost for how much it will cost to move yourself and your family, which may exceed a fixed dollar amount. Then, you can negotiate to have the middle offer accepted by both parties to ensure that all of your items are moved. Quite honestly, how would we know if $5,000 was enough to move your entire

apartment from Los Angeles to Washington, DC, for example?

> *Power Move #41 - Negotiate to obtain three quotes for the costs of your relocation and agree to accept the middle quote.*

> Red Flag: The provision of relocation expenses is now more frequently being tied to a minimum time commitment. Meaning if you leave the practice prior to the specified term, you may have to pay back some portion of these relocation expenses. Hence, this becomes more of a relocation LOAN vs. a bonus. In addition, please check the tax implications of having your relocation expenses covered.

Note: I often hear doctors express disdain for the employer for not informing us about the details surrounding our tax liability or other issues.

- o First, it is NOT the employer's responsibility to educate us about the business or financial aspects of being employed.
- o Secondly, the employer may not actually know every tax implication as they apply to your life.

It is our responsibility to become better informed with the help of our team of advisors so that we can make better decisions and live our best lives.

OTHER VARIABLE COMPENSATION COMPONENTS, MISCELLANEOUS EXPENSES:

Additional compensation components to be negotiated could include:

o   Association Membership Dues and Licensing Fees
o   Equipment – Provision of a cell phone, computer, etc.
o   Parking – Parking pass or coverage of parking costs
o   Travel – Travel reimbursements may be provided, especially
    if travel is required between two or more locations

Reimbursements from the practice in accordance with IRS rules will be identified, especially regarding daily food and travel reimbursement costs, aka a per diem. These reimbursements often include Continuing medical education expenses to attend courses or conferences.

PART 2 – UNDERSTANDING CURRENT COMPENSATION MODELS

This chapter serves a brief tutorial on the relatively complex subject of doctor compensation models, which most commonly include:

o   Guaranteed Salary
o   RVU Productivity-Based
o   Quality-Based
o   Net Revenue-Based
o   Income Guarantee

Now in my mind, this should not be as complex of a subject as it is, but because it is complex, it is worth exploring the foundation of what the different doctor compensation models look like in as much detail as possible. Thus, the goal of this chapter is to help doctors understand:

o   The varying types of compensation models
o   How to estimate annual compensation income
o   What relevant questions should be asked on a routine basis
    to help determine your compensation
o   Recommended action steps to proactively monitor your
    compensation

This chapter is for new doctors or doctors early in their career who are moving into a six-figure salary compensation for the first or second time since leaving residency. It's also for doctors who may be transitioning from one type of practice to another so that you are clear about what to expect.

For example, I worked with a doctor-scientist whose priority it was to start her own research lab while also seeing patients clinically. So, she negotiated a part of her compensation package to include the provision of physical lab space, equipment, and a research team equipping her with the capacity to submit additional grants to obtain future funding to support her lab moving forward. Just imagine if this doctor had only focused on the salary aspect of her contract, then she would have missed the opportunity to negotiate for the resources to support her research objectives. Ultimately, she was able to satisfy her needs and her wants in her contract negotiations.

Breaking Down Physician Compensation Models

Depending on what type of practice you are joining, the model used to determine your compensation will vary. The following compensation models might vary based on the organization. Unfortunately, these compensation models share a commonality of being more complex than they are simple to understand, which is why we are taking me time to review these compensation models.

GUARANTEED SALARY

First, let's start with the guaranteed salary compensation model. This model states that starting from year one, a doctor's annual base salary will remain the same in subsequent years two and three, etc. This constant annual compensation may contingent on the doctor satisfying the requirements of working full-time, which is commonly referred to as a Full-Time Equivalent (FTE) position.

> **Full-time equivalents** (FTEs) are units measuring work done defined by a certain length of time for a full-time position.

For example, the number of hours for most employed positions equates to a person working 40 hours per week. Therefore, this employee would expect to work 8 hours per day for 5 days per week, which equates to 40 hours/week = one FTE. Contrastingly, one Full-Time Equivalent position for doctors averages between 50-60 hours per week. This means that the expectation is that a full-time job for a doctor might equate to 20 additional hours on top of what's customary for a non-professional or non-medical professional.

There are a few additional definitions that are important to explore at this point include:

A **salary** is the type of compensation that is usually assigned at the professional or management level. A salary is a set amount paid over a specific interval of time, which may be on a bi-weekly or monthly basis.

This is different from a wage, which is an hourly amount paid to an employee. The amount of time worked is regulated, and overtime is generally compensated with additional hourly wages.

IMPORTANT: Doctor-employees are categorized as "exempt" employees from overtime laws because they are viewed as professionals and are in management. Physicians can expect to work a full-time equivalent or more and not anticipate or expect to be paid overtime.

Overtime pay for eligible employees is strictly regulated and must be monitored closely and documented by the practice or by the health care system. Violation of overtime wages can land any company or organization in big trouble. If you run a practice and have hourly workers make sure you have a standardized process for monitoring their time worked, so any overtime can be paid accordingly, routinely, and on time.

Alternatively, it is possible to negotiate working less than one FTE. For example, a doctor could work 60%(0.6) or 80% (0.8) FTE, if your preference is to work part-time. As a result, your salary would then be calculated by multiplying the salary for one FTE times 0.6 to yield the annual pay.

For example, if the annual guaranteed salary for one FTE = $200,000, then the annual base salary for a doctor working 0.6 FTEs is:

$$\$200,000 \times 0.6 = \$120,000 \text{ annual base salary}$$

One additional question that should be asked is regarding employee benefits. Each organization will indicate the MINIMUM number of FTEs that must be worked in order to receive employee benefits. This information can usually be found in the Employee Handbook developed by the employer.

Guaranteed Salary Illustration

The guaranteed salary in which your base salary remains the same on an annualized basis provides you with that stability compensation model.

Take this table, for example. The annual guaranteed salary for this position is $200,000. This is the gross salary amount, and that number would be constant from year to year. This amount usually is not based on how productive you are, i.e. how many patients you see, how many procedures you perform.

	Year 1	Year 2	Year 3
Guaranteed Salary	200,000	200,000	200,000

Figure 13 – Guaranteed Salary Comparison Table

Whether you have negotiated additional variable compensation components or not, knowing that our annual base pay will remain constant can provide a level of stability thereby allowing strategic financial and life plans to be developed. Certainly, annual cost of living raises should be inquired about, as well, but knowing the base pay rate can provide a source of potential stability.

> Red Flag: Please note that although this base compensation amount is set to be constant irrespective of your productivity, we must always remember that this is business and that your productivity is still being monitored when you are receiving a guaranteed salary. Therefore, I will caution every doctor to:
>
> o avoid becoming complacent by doing the minimum amount of work possible. Practices have been known to reduce one's annual base salary if the physician is not generating enough revenue to cover their overhead costs.
> o Monitor your productivity even if you are receiving a guaranteed salary to ensure that your base salary will not be compromised.
> o Then, review and compare your own productivity data with that of the practice/employer to confirm that your productivity is being measured accurately, so that there are no discrepancies when annual compensation/budget reviews take place.

Doc: What if I am so productive that I am exceeding the minimum productivity requirements? Could I actually be generating more than the base salary that is being offered?

Dr. Bonnie: Great questions! Now, if you find that your productivity is far exceeding the amount reflected in your base pay, the option to renegotiate your guaranteed salary to a productivity-based compensation model may exist. By all means, negotiate for the model that converts all of your hard work into dollars.

This leads us to our next compensation model.

RVU PRODUCTIVITY- BASED COMPENSATION MODEL

A productivity-based compensation model, which says that you will be compensated based on how productive you are, i.e. how many patients you see or how many procedures you perform, both of which are measured in Relative Value Units (RVUs) you generate.

Wait? What is an RVU?

An RVU is a relative value unit, which translates the relative amount of work required for the doctor to take care of a patient for diagnosis and procedure. It is the relative value of the amount of work required for that doctor to render care to that patient.

RVUs are broken down into 3 components:

- o Physicians work RVUs (wRVUs)
- o Practice Expenses RVUs
- o Practice Liability RVUs

For the sake of this discussion, we will only be referring to wRVUs.

How are Relative Value Units calculated?

The Centers for Medicare and Medicaid Services (CMS) has a list of the standard number of RVUs that are assigned to the different evaluation and management codes, as well as to each International Classification of Diseases, 10th edition (ICD-10) codes, as well as to the Current Procedural Terminology (CPT) codes[8].

CMS provides a guide for practices and hospitals to use in order to calculate RVUs. However, EACH PRACTICE/EMPLOYER CAN CHOOSE TO CALCULATE RVUs DIFFERENTLY.

According to physician coding specialist, Dr. Charlotte Akor, it is mandatory for each doctor to understand[9]:

- o How RVUs are generated in the hospital/practice setting?

- o How many RVUs on average are assigned to every Evaluation & Management (E & M), ICD-10, and CPT code?
- o What RVU conversion factor is being used to calculate my compensation?
- o What is the formula being used to calculate my compensation?
- o When do I receive credit for the RVUs that I generate?
- o Upon work performed or upon collection of revenue?
- o Will I be penalized if there is a problem in the billing and collections?

The complexity of the patient's diagnosis, as well as the complexity of the care rendered, work to determine the RVUs, but this gets complicated because there are thousands of ICD-10 and CPT codes that are used in the coding and billing process.

For example, a patient that has hypertension and diabetes who requires cholecystectomy will generate a higher level of RVUs that will be generated versus a patient who comes in for a routine physical with no PMH.

> *Power Move #42 - All doctors should do their own coding! Take a coding course on an annual basis to understand medical coding and billing for your specialty, especially if you are in your first 3 years of practice.*

There are several reasons for this vehement recommendation:

1. The law states that it is the doctor's responsibility to select the billing code that most accurately reflects the services that were provided during a patient encounter.
   a. Inaccurate coding, intentional or unintentional, is a serious offense that can easily be identified during audits.
   b. Do not allow an employer to direct you or their staff to up code (increase the level of services to collect more money) your patient services. This is billing

fraud, which can result in criminal charges being brought against you.

2. Your medical license on the line every time you submit a claim. When we bill third-party payors, we are certifying that everything that is being billed is accurate. Many doctors have gone to jail for fraudulent billing practices, whether they were aware of what was going on or not, because you are the responsible party for this by law.

3. No one knows better than you, Doc, about what transpired in the exam room between you and your patient. Hence, the most accurate description of the diagnosis and procedures can and should be captured by you. Certainly, your coder can double-check your codes and modifiers, but you cannot expect anyone to do this part of your job better than you will, especially in a productivity-based compensation model. You want to ensure maximum and accurate charge-capture in the billing process.

THE RVU CONVERSION FACTOR

Not only do you need to know how many RVUs you're going to generate, but you must also know what your RVU conversion factor is and how many RVUs are being assigned to your specific services rendered.

Again, I recommend meeting with the practice administrator at least quarterly to reconcile your productivity data with that of the practice's data set and to build an understanding of how RVUs are calculated in the practice.

It is up to you to build an understanding of RVUs and the use of the RVU-based system in your particular specialty and region for your particular type of practice. I highly recommend the reference book, Coding and Billing Mastery by Dr. Charlotte Akor, in order to build a baseline understanding of all of the above.

A COMPENSATION CASE STUDY

In Figure 14, a doctor is offered a position under an RVU-based compensation model starting with:

- an annual base salary guarantee of $200,000 for each of the first two years, Year 1 & Year 2
- a compensation model converting to an RVU productivity-based model requiring a productivity minimum of 4000 RVUs in Year 3

RVU -Based Compensation Model
RVU minimum requirement/year = 4000 RVUs/year

	Year 1	Year 2	Year 3	Year 4
RVUs generated/yr	2800	3500		
Base Compensation	$200,000	$200,000		

Figure 14 – RVU Compensation Model, Part 1

In Years 1 and 2, you have generated 2800 and 3500 RVUs, respectively. For each year, you have also received the $200,000 guaranteed annual salary. So far, so good.

Doc: Why do practices provide a guaranteed salary in the first 1-2 years?

Dr. Bonnie: For the following reasons, just to name a few:

- It also takes 60- 120 days for the doctor to become credentialed with their hospitals or medical centers and with each of the third-party payers. During this waiting period, the doctor cannot submit any claims, therefore the practice provides a salary during the down period.

- o Practices understand that it takes time (6-18 months) for doctors to build up the number of patients in their patient panel and to reach a level of workflow efficiency into their daily practices.
- o Training of new physicians and the recruitment of new patients customarily take 6-9 months or more, so the standard practice is to guarantee a salary for that period.

As previously stated, the number of RVUs that you generate in year one of your Foundational Contract (see Chapter $) will be used to calculate your base salary in your productivity-based contract, which is usually your Renewal Contract.

VERY IMPORTANT: As stated in the section on Guaranteed Salaries earlier in this chapter, always monitor and document your own productivity (the number of patients seen in every clinical setting, along with their respective E & M, ICD-10 and CPT codes) especially in year 1 of this RVU-based compensation model.

Back to the Case Study:

Then, in Year 3, your productivity stays at 3500 RVUs instead of increasing to the minimum productivity requirement of 4000 RVUs. This subsequently negatively affects your annual base compensation. See Figure 15.

RVU -Based Compensation Model
RVU minimum requirement/year = 4000 RVUs/year

	Year 1	Year 2	Year 3	Year 4
RVUs generated/yr	2800	3500	3500	
Base Compensation	$200,000	$200,000	$175,000	
			-$25,000	

Figure 15 – RVU Compensation Model, Part 2

Why? Well, three things happened here:

1. Your productivity in Years 1-2 was being monitored, so essentially your Year 3 salary was going to be based on your productivity in Year 2 even though you were still receiving a guaranteed salary.
2. The RVU calculation based on 3500 annual RVUs equates to $175,000 in annual compensation, which we could have discovered if we had been meeting with our administrator routinely in Year 2.
3. You did not know that you were only generating 3500 vs. 4000 RVUs in Year 3.

This is when I receive calls from alarmed docs who didn't know that their annual salary was about to be cut by $25,000, which is more than one month's pay.

Yikes! Any drop in salary truly hurts, and my heart hurts when I hear stories like this from my doctor colleagues.

> ### *Power Move #43* - *Maximize & DOCUMENT your productivity during your foundational years even while you are on a guaranteed salary!*

So now that your salary has dropped secondary to you not having met your productivity minimum, what are your options:

a. Document your productivity weekly and verify your numbers with administrators monthly
b. Meet with your administrators to find out what you can do to increase your productivity
c. Meet with your administrators to explore what they are willing to do to help you increase your productivity
d. a, b, c

In contrast, there's nothing worse than working our tails off seeing patients around the clock, just to find out that our productivity has not been accurately recorded by the practice, hospital, or medical center. Listen...no one has a greater interest in making sure that your productivity is accurately recorded than you do. No one!

Otherwise, you are just working for free, and we are not going to work for free anymore!

Now, let's take a look at what happens in Year 4 once you have increased your productivity.

RVU -Based Compensation Model
RVU minimum requirement/year = 4000 RVUs/year

	Year 1	Year 2	Year 3	Year 4
RVUs generated/yr	2800	3500	3500	4500
Base Compensation	$200,000	$200,000	$175,000	$225,000
			-$25,000	+$25,000

Figure 16 – RVU Compensation Model, Part 3

In Year 4, your productivity increased to 4500 RVUs with a resulting productivity bonus of $25,000. See Figure 16. #awesome

Understandably, these variations in compensation can serve as an extreme source of anxiety and stress in the midst of our busy clinical and personal lives, and this issue lies at the core of over half of the distress calls that I receive from doctors across the country.

Why? Because many of us do not understand the productivity-based model, we are often caught off-guard. Being notified about a five or six-figure decrease in salary would raise anyone's stress level. So, let's prevent it!

The important point to understand about productivity-based compensation models is that your compensation will likely vary because it depends on your productivity, which may vary due to things you may or may not control.

Here are some examples that I have heard from physicians over the years regarding aspects of practice that influence a productivity-based salary:

- o the practice plans on hiring 3 additional docs in your specialty, then this may dilute the number of patients that might be referred to see you
- o the practice opens an additional location where the patient volume is low
- o the practice has recently lost 3 physicians, which would leave you in a situation with too many patients which could lead to burnout if there is not a plan to hire additional physicians
- o the practice does not provide adequate clinical support, i.e. medical assistants or technicians

Therefore, upon receipt of an employment contract that includes a productivity-based compensation offer, be sure to pose the following critical questions to the practice to determine whether the minimum number of RVUs is achievable, including:

- o How many RVUs are the doctors generating in this practice who are in my specialty and working in this office? How many years have they been in practice?
- o How many patients on average clinically have to be seen either in the office or in an operative or procedure setting in order for you to generate the 4,800 RVUs per year?
- o Will there be enough infrastructure and capacity in place in order to generate the minimum RVUs per year, such as the necessary support staff and number of offices needed to meet the RVU minimum?
- o What is the RVU conversion factor used for our specialty, particular region, health system, and practice?
- o May I see an illustration of how the RVU values are calculated in this potential practice?
- o Does the practice have any expansion/acquisition plans that may affect my position?
- o Also assess/research physician turnover/retention in the practice to gauge the culture of the practice as being physician-friendly or not. This is not a question that should be posed to the practice leadership, but one that should be asked strategically and with tact of the current physicians

and staff perhaps during a site visit or during follow-up interviews.

Finally, we want to do our due diligence by researching the answers from our specialty societies, within the local hospitals/medical centers and with our doctor colleagues who have recently transitioned into practice. Online references such as Merritt Hawkins, compensation data from the AAMCs, even physician survey data from sources like Medscape, can inform us of what to expect regarding productivity and compensation norms.

In conclusion, we must SIP to Success™ by planning to minimize these variables in our compensation by making these critical Power Moves while we are in practice:

Power Move #44 - Intentionally document your productivity, i.e., the number, ICD-10, CPT codes for every patient that you see in every clinical setting.

Power Move #45 - Proactively communicate with administrators to review and verify the documentation of your productivity and the accurate calculation of your RVU calculations.

Power Move #46 - Strategically work within your practice to ensure that your productivity is maximized.

Power Move #47 - Strategically work with your financial advisor to develop a budget that can provide financial security in the event that your productivity and hence your compensation varies.

Because of the aforementioned potential uncertainties and considering the levels of financial investment and sacrifice that we've made in our careers, not knowing how much money we're going to bring home can be very stressful and destabilizing.

However, we now know what we can do to get in front of the RV-based compensation model. Let's go!

QUALITY-BASED PRODUCTIVITY

Quality metrics are being integrated into the calculation of doctors' compensation more frequently over the past 10 years. This is undoubtedly an effort from the federal government to incentivize providers to improve the quality and delivery of care.

Specific quality measures are determined by each practice or employer. It is important that you understand which quality metrics apply to the position that you are considering.

Here is an example of a set of quality measurements in Figure 17:

Sample Quality Metrics

Performance standards shall be as follows:

Annual Quality Measurements

Participant shall receive annual incentive salary of Five Hundred Dollars ($500.00) for each quality measure, if the required compliance level for the associated measure has been met.

For patients requiring procedures, Participant will be measured on the following Measurements:

  Measure 1 – Prophylactic Antibiotic Received within One Hour prior to Medical or Surgical Procedure

  Measure 2 – Appropriate Antibiotic Selection for Patients with Medical or Surgical Procedures

  Measure 3 – Prophylactic Antibiotics Discontinued Within 24 Hours After Procedure or Surgery End Time

  Measure 4 – Hospital Acquired Procedural/Surgical Infections

In order to be eligible to receive an incentive payment, Participant must achieve at least the following compliance percentage for each measure:

  Measure 1, 2, and 3- 100% compliance

  Measure 4 - Year 2 Improvement or no change in Measure from Year 1

    - Year 3 Improvement or no change in Measure from Year 2

Figure 17 – Sample Quality Metrics

According to this illustration, the doctor shall receive an annual incentive salary of $500 for each quality measure achieved, if the required compliance level for the associated measure has been met.

In Year 1, quality measures #1, #2 and #3 must be met, and in Year 2 and in Year 3, all of four of the measures must be met or improved upon. If all of the measures are met, the doctor would be eligible to receive $500 for each of the four quality measures, which would equate to $2,000 to be included in your salary payments.

Now that we understand how to achieve these measures, we have to evaluate the feasibility of the quality metrics.

A closer look at these requirements reveals that there is only quality measure, #2, that is directly tied to the doctor's delivery of care. Certainly, appropriate antibiotic selection is absolutely a care measure for which the doctor should be primarily. However, in review of measures #1 and #3, satisfactory compliance will depend on the entire healthcare team being compliant with the timely administration or discontinuation of antibiotics. In addition, measure #4 is an outcome measure of the presence of hospital-acquired infection, which is dependent on the entire healthcare team and environment. Therefore, it is up to us to ask enough questions regarding whether and how the entire healthcare team has been trained in order to meet these quality measures.

> Red Flag - In some systems, the doctor's compensation can also be reduced by the quality metrics by failing to meet designated quality

At the end of the day, it is important that you understand the expectations that you are being incentivized to meet, but you have to understand whether these are actually achievable or not, and what your final compensation payment will be with and without the quality metrics model.

QUALITY-BASED METRICS CASE STUDY

Quality-Based Metrics Compensation Model

RVU minimum requirement/year = 4000 RVUs/year

	Year 1	Year 2	Year 3	Year 4
RVUs generated/yr	2800	3500	3500	4000
Base Compensation	$200,000	$200,000	$175,000	$200,000
Incentive Pay	$2,000	$2,000	$2,000	$2,000

Figure 18 – Quality-Based Metrics Compensation Model

Now, upon further review of the contract offered to our doctor who is on an RVU-based compensation model from the previous case, we discover that the requirement to satisfy quality measures is also built into the compensation package.

Fortunately, in each year of practice, the doctor met with 100% compliance for the quality measures and received the incentive pay of $2,000 every year for meeting those quality measures on an annual basis. #strongwork

NET REVENUE-BASED COMPENSATION MODEL

A compensation model based on net revenue generated by the physician is actually a newer compensation model that I've seen evolve over the last few years.

In a net revenue-based compensation model, our initial questions to the practice should be:

o What is net revenue?
o How is net revenue calculated?

Remember, every word being used in your contract is there for a reason. If there's something you do not understand, then you have to ask.

The answers to these questions must begin by understanding the gross revenue and the expenses for the practice, e.g.,

Gross Revenue - Expenses = Net Revenue

It is the net revenue that the doctor's salary will be calculated from. Yet, this brings up two important sets of questions:

o Let's understand that the doctor has some influence on the gross revenue that he or she generates from seeing patients, however this equation does not clarify whether this is gross revenue billed or collected.
o The physician has less, if any, influence over the practice's expenses which includes its overhead costs for payroll, salaries, utilities, etc. This is important because if a practice poorly manages its expenses which would be subtracted from our gross revenue generation, that our net revenue/compensation will be negatively impacted.

Let's dig a little deeper by reviewing sample contract language that outlines the details of this net-revenue based compensation offer for additional answers:

o The Practice would employ the Physician full-time for a term of five (5) years.
o The Practice would provide the Physician with a guaranteed minimum base salary for clinical, professional work – only as follows:
  o Year 1 – greater of $195,000 base guarantee or net revenue-based compensation
  o Years 2-5 – net revenue-based compensation

o The NET revenue-based compensation is based on actual collections for services personally performed by the doctor minus overhead and any deductions you may have selected, like health insurance payments.
o It is a nationally recognized approach to quantifying productivity, and it is commonly used as a basis for compensating doctors.
o The formula for doctor compensation is a percent of actual collections received for services performed by the Physician.
o The percent of collections would be 48%.

To understand how the net revenue is calculated, the contract says that,

o The NET revenue-based compensation is based on actual collections for services personally performed by the Physician minus overhead.

Another important detail is:

o The formula for doctor compensation is a percent of actual collections received for services performed by the Physician.

Finally, the contract also states that the percent of actual collections that will translate into the doctor's salary is 48%.

The next most important questions must be:

o How is the doctor's overhead calculated? Which expenses are included in overhead?
o How accurate are the practice's collections? What percent of the billing does the practice collect?

The interesting thing about this model is that as of now, we still do not know what the physician's annual salary will be. Yikes!

Here, we see that in Year 1, there is a guaranteed salary of $195,000 or net-revenue-based compensation, whichever is greater. So, let's assume in Year 1 that the doctor receives the guaranteed salary of $195,000.

Then in Year 2, Dr. X generates and bills for $500,000. The accuracy of the employer's collections is measured by its collections ratio, which is 60%. This means that the practice collects 60% of all of the revenue that is collectible based on the doctor's billings.

Taking a look at the correlating equation, the practice will collect 60% of the $500,000 billed by the doctor, which amounts to $300,000.

Employer's collection ratio is 60% = ($500,000 x 0.6) = $300,000

Thus, $300,000 is the amount of the actual collections based on the doctor's billings.

Since the doctor's percent of collections equals 48%, the doctor's take-home salary is equivalent to:

$$\$300,000 \times .48 = \$144,000$$

Based on this net-revenue-based formula, the doctor would generate the following compensation in Years 1 & 2:

Net Revenue -Based Compensation Model

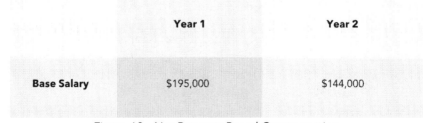

	Year 1	Year 2
Base Salary	$195,000	$144,000

Figure 19 – Net-Revenue Based Compensation

For Educational Purposes Only. Not Intended as Legal Advice.

The resulting compensation in Year 2 is almost 25% less than it is in Year 1 based on the contract. It is up to you to decide whether you and your family can manage this level of compensation variability. As noted here, the variability is largely based on the practice's failure to efficiently collect the revenue that the physician generated, as evidenced by the 60% collections ratio. The converse could hold as well, if the practice had a 90% collections ratio then the net-revenue collected based on the physician's billing would be

$$\$500,000 \times .9 = \$480,000$$

When multiplied by the physician's percent of collections of 48%,

$$\$480,000 \times .48 = \$216,000$$

This is certainly a better outcome than in the former illustration, but the point here is that we

Red Flag: In this scenario, transparency on behalf of the practice is critical. If the practice cannot or will not share their collections ratio, then you may want to reconsider joining this particular practice. Simply put, a practice should know how well it is collecting revenue eligible for collection, and optimal collection ratios hover closer to 90% vs. 50-60%.

Thus, it would behoove every doctor to make sure that when you see this type of compensation model that you actually move very, very slowly through dissecting exactly what the potential compensation numbers will look like for you. Based on the historical numbers that the practice can provide, the employer's collections ratio, and how well they manage their overhead costs, you should be able to engage this informed-decision making process that is data-driven. This is the goal!

INCOME GUARANTEE

The last compensation model that we want to discuss is the income guarantee. Earlier in chapter 9, I discussed a guaranteed salary. An income guarantee is different, although the verbiage sounds similar. An income guarantee is also known as a hospital assistance or a relocation assistance compensation package.

Have you seen physician employment advertisements that tout really high dollar amounts, e.g. $500,000 for primary care physicians or close to $1million dollars for specialists? Many of these advertisements are for income guarantee arrangements.

These income guarantees are used to recruit doctors to practice in their communities, often rural or underserved areas. During the typical 12-24 month term of an income guarantee, the local hospital and/or practice will advance, or LOAN, a specified amount of money to the physician in order to:

- o allow the physician to build a new practice in the community
- o cover the physician's salary as determined by the fair market value for physician salaries in that region that are specialty-specific

The second part of this arrangement includes a forgiveness period. This financial support then either can be forgiven by the hospital with a time commitment from the physician, typically in a 2:1 ratio, e.g. the physician agrees to work in the community for 2 years for every year of financial support. If for whatever reason, the doctor does not continue working in the community for the specified loan forgiveness period, the amount of the income guarantee usually must be repaid in full with interest and often other stipulations, which are often quite unfavorable to the physician.

Several of my doctor colleagues have entered into these arrangements over the years without a full understanding of what would be required and the subsequent consequences of not being able to fulfill the time obligation or not being able to build a profitable practice in a short period or time (with no business experience). The consequences for not doing so can be horrific, so I recommend the following:

- o If you are being recruited to set up a new practice, confirm whether this is an income guarantee arrangement FIRST
- o Next, get a lawyer! The financial and legal intricacies of these arrangements are extremely complex, especially because of the amounts of monies that are involved, and these arrangements must not violate
  - o Federal Stark Laws
  - o Anti-kickback Statutes
  - o IRS private benefit guidance, for non-profit organizations
- o Always read the contract documents in full, as there will likely be 2-3 sets of documents involved in this arrangement, including:
  - o physician services agreement, possibly between multiple parties
  - o equipment leases if applicable
  - o separate loan document called a PROMISSORY NOTE (Remember, promissory notes are loan documents that outline the financial details, i.e. loan repayment schedules, principal and interest, penalties and guarantees, that we are committing to, so we must carefully review these documents with our lawyer, financial advisor and tax accountant BEFORE ever signing a promissory note.)
- o Be sure that you have prepared yourself to build a business, i.e. practice, while simultaneously building a new practice, which the majority of physicians have not been taught to do.

Remember the old saying, that if it looks too good to be true, it probably is! So, unless you are a super, sub-sub specialized physician, salary offers approximating a million dollars should prompt caution and further investigation. This may actually be an income guarantee. However, if you prepare properly, have a trusted team of advisors and the environment is one where you guarantee that you can build a thriving business, then this arrangement could work for you.

CHAPTER SUMMARY

POWER MOVES

o It is important for physicians to read through the contract for ourselves, before reviewing it with our team of advisors. The more we practice reading contracts, the less daunting they will become.

o Take heed of the top 5 contract terms that all physicians should be aware of:

o Do not be wooed by the salary being offered in the contract as the top priority

o Instead, let's do our due diligence to understand the fair market value for physician compensation for a specific region and for our specialty

o Understand the specifics of the compensation model that is being proposed for your position

RED FLAGS

o Always read every page, exhibit and/or appendix of your contract. This is especially important if you see a PROMISSORY NOTE, which is a loan document. Then, stop and review this document with your team of advisors, because we likely want to eliminate increasing our debt burden after so many years of training and with existing educational debt.

o If the proposed salary for a new position is extremely high, then this may be an income guarantee arrangement. Be aware!

HOMEWORK

o Take time to do your due diligence in researching physician compensation values for your specialty, geographic region and number of years in practice

o Alert your team of advisors that you will need their support in order to facilitate having your contract reviewed by each of them before entering contract negotiations

o Work with your financial advisor and tax accountant to graph your anticipated income and expenses for the term of your contract. This is called a pro forma, a projected budget that will allow you to make the best informed decision based on data, instead of one that is based on fear or desperation.

REFERENCES

8. www.CMS.gov
9. Akor, Charlotte. Coding and Billing Mastery. 2019

NOTES

_____

_____

_____

_____

_____

_____

_____

_____

_____

_____

_____

_____

_____

_____

_____

_____

_____

_____

Chapter 10

TOP 5 NEGOTIATION MISTAKES DOCTORS MAKE

Doc: *Dr. Bonnie, I just signed my contract.*

Dr. Bonnie: *Congratulations! How did your negotiations go?*

Doc: *What negotiations? I didn't negotiate at all. I just signed the contract to get it over with.*

Dr. Bonnie: *(Silence)*

In the current healthcare environment, negotiating is critical because of my current mantra, which is:

"Doctors are in healthcare.
Healthcare is a business.
Therefore, doctors are in business."
Bonnie Simpson Mason

After completing my residency training, I joined a private practice in orthopedics. At the time, I was given the opportunity to become the physician executive and lead administrator in that practice. In a very short period of time, it became clear to me that understanding contracts and negotiations was a fundamental skill that I must learn and become more comfortable with as a practicing physician. Certainly, making these critical decisions made me very nervous and uncomfortable on a daily basis. Despite these feelings of discomfort, I emphatically recommend that all physicians, both current and future, learn about the business of medicine, especially contracts and negotiations even while in medical school and residency training. We now know that our lives depend on it.

In this chapter, we will review:

- o common negotiating landmines and mistakes
- o what good signs and positive indicators in negotiations look like
- o major Red Flags

These are actually mental landmines that we tell ourselves during times of transition and negotiation, which should be absolutely avoided. These mental landmines can lead to common mistakes when negotiating.

Top Negotiating Mistakes Physicians Make

Mistake #1 - We fail to shift our mindset from a student or trainee to the real world of practicing medicine, and many of us just don't negotiate at all.

Our first step in learning how to successfully negotiate is to master our mindset. Throughout medical school and training, we have been taught to be satisfied when we've received a medical school acceptance or when we've matched into residency/fellowship. Certainly, there was no negotiating in either of these processes, so there's no surprise that we are neither familiar with nor are comfortable with the thought of having to negotiate for everything that we need and want once we move into practice.

Instead, we must consider embracing the following thoughts:

1. Negotiating is expected in business, and since healthcare is a business, we are expected to negotiate.
2. When we do our research, we will understand our value/our worth. Then, we can confidently negotiate for parity in compensation based on data and not based on speculation.

> *Power Move #48 - I am changing my mindset around negotiating.*
> *I can do this!*

I have heard firsthand many doctors say that they don't want to negotiate. In fact, over 50% of the physicians whom I have mentored and coached admit that they did not negotiate their employment contracts at all.

Clearly, we now understand that NOT negotiating is NOT an option, let's think of negotiations as having critical conversations. Ahhh, doesn't that sound better?

Given the fact that we have critical conversations every day with our patients, building partnerships with them to help achieve better health outcomes, we have to get into the practice of having critical conversations around business and finance. We can absolutely have critical conversations with our potential employer where we ask the hard questions because that's what business and adulting require.

Next, we can prepare for negotiations in partnership with our health law attorney and our financial advisors to help us develop a negotiation strategy. This should be followed-up with role-playing or having a sample script for negotiating will help us build our confidence levels.

> **Power Move #49** - *Consult our advisors* → *Collect our data* →
> *Build a Negotiation Strategy* → *Practice* → *Negotiate* → *Win!*

Mistake #2 - We don't pursue multiple employment opportunities.

We can position ourselves most favorably during any negotiation by having leverage. One way to build leverage is to weigh multiple employment positions simultaneously, and not just focusing on only one position.

Comparing multiple (2-3) opportunities allows us to evaluate multiple compensation packages that are being offered in the market. We can then compare apples to apples and use favorable aspects from other offers to negotiate for similar terms in the position that we are leaning towards the most.

> For example, let's consider employment opportunities in Practice A and Practice B. Practice B is in your preferred location with one office and is offering a salary that is below the 25th percentile range for new physicians. However, Practice B is offering a salary that is in the 45th percentile, but requires the physician to work at multiple locations, which is less favorable for you and your family. Here, you could leverage this information and negotiate for a salary that is closer to the 45th percentile based on what the fair market is offering.

Just remember that we have compared multiple options before when applying to medical and to residency programs. We always reviewed more than one school or program. Now, we get to apply the same process in the real world. Please see the <u>Power Moves Employment Options Tracker</u> in Section 2 of your Power Moves Workbook, which will enable you to capture and compare the details of the employment options that you are considering.

Mistake #3 – We don't negotiate person to person.

A critical negotiation mistake we make is that we don't negotiate person to person. Negotiations, aka critical conversations, yield the best results for both parties when negotiations take place person to person.

Ideally, we should also negotiate on our own behalf first, instead of engaging our attorney to do so. Moreover, I strongly recommend doing so face to face, person to person if possible. Certainly, if you're negotiating for a position long distance, then multiple face-to-face conversations are unlikely to happen. However, most negotiations should take place verbally over the phone rather than having the primary mode of communication take place via email or text.

Overall, negotiating is an exercise in relationship building, and we want to build this professional relationship in a way where you can pick up as many emotional and physical cues as possible. The most effective way to build any relationship is by speaking to the person.

I have learned firsthand that using text or email as the primary mode for negotiating allows for contact avoidance. It is actually quite easy for someone to type "no" in an email vs. discussing the reasons for turning down your request in person or over the phone. Text and emails during negotiations also leave significant room for misinterpretation, whereas person to person negotiation often lead to resolution faster because both parties are humanized.

> **Power Move #50** - *Remember that negotiating is part of a relationship-building process. So start building this relationship by negotiating for yourself and do so face-to-face, or at least person to person.*

Mistake #4 – We fail to document.

In the context of negotiations, ALL conversations that transpire during negotiations should be documented via email that can be referred to at a later date as a record of verbal commitments. This is the Intentional Documentation aspect of the SIP to Success Strategy.

How and what to document:

Immediately following a critical conversation, follow-up with an email, which is date and time-stamped, within 24 hours to the other party.

Your follow-up email should include:

o Thanking the person(s) for their time and for the conversation first and foremost
o Reiterating the specific points that were reviewed during the conversation, along with the details of any agreements that were made during the conversation
o Requesting a time for your next follow-up conversation and recapping next steps for each party

These are the three things that should be in every follow-up email during a negotiation, as a point of reference and to create a paper trail. This ensures that both parties are clear about what was discussed and to make sure that everyone is on the same page.

In addition, documenting points of agreement during negotiations is critical, just as documenting our productivity while we are in practice can equate to revenue that can be lost or gained. In short, documentation = dollars, and your documentation serves as proof of your productivity, which you can leverage in future negotiations.

Just as we documented our case logs in residency, we can form the habit of documenting the details of our patient encounters in every setting to accurately capture our productivity.

> *Power Move #51* - *Be intentional about documenting your critical conversations during negotiations (and in practice for that matter) by sending a follow-up email recap to the person with whom you are negotiating. This provides a date and time stamp along with a written record of what was covered and agreed/disagreed on during the conversation, which may be helpful for future reference.*

Mistake #5 – We don't practice negotiating before negotiating.

The next contract mistake we make is that we don't practice negotiating prior to having our actual critical conversations with our respective employers.

In order to decrease our anxiety while treading in these unfamiliar waters, I am encouraging every Doc to practice negotiating via role-playing before going into negotiations with:

- o   A physician mentor
- o   A colleague who has recently transitioned into practice
- o   A person who is well-versed in business
- o   Your health law attorney and financial advisor

> **Power Move #52** - *Consult our advisors → Collect our data → Build a Negotiation Strategy→ Practice → Negotiate → Win!*

This can be compared to not practicing for our medical school or residency interviews ahead of time. Each of us has either been the person who did not practice our interviewing skills ahead of time, or we have been the person interviewing someone who has failed to prepare and practice. Let's not be that person now. We know better.

Bonus Mistake - Many times, we are unwilling to walk away from a negotiation.

I spoke about leverage earlier in this chapter, because weighing more than one opportunity in any situation gives us the most leverage possible. Having multiple opportunities also provides us with options, so that we don't just have to take a single offer that is presented to us. We can actually walk away, turn down, kindly decline an offer if negotiations take a turn for the worst.

One option is not an option at all; this is an obligation.

Examples of negotiations going poorly include:

- o Communications that are delayed, poor responsiveness
- o Lack of flexibility when negotiating common aspects of the practice
- o Lack of transparency or clarity when asking employers to be specific
- o Lack of cordiality

In these ways and more, the tenor of our negotiations can give us a hint about the culture of the organization, whether it is physician-supportive or not, and whether this might be a good fit for us or not. Every position is not the best position for us, so if we find that it is not, then we have to be willing to pursue our other options.

CHAPTER SUMMARY

POWER MOVES

- o Shift our mindset into one that is empowered through education and collaboration with our team of advisors.
- o Always negotiate AFTER devising a data-driven strategy.
- o Consult with your team of advisors as soon as you identify the top 3 practices that you may consider joining.
- o Practice. Practice. Practice. (Review this chapter for details)
- o Document. Document. Document. (Documentation = $$$)

RED FLAGS

- o These are fundamental landmines that we can all proactively avoid when negotiations are pending.

HOMEWORK

- o Take 48 hours to observe when you are negotiating, aka having critical conversations, in your everyday life.
- o Then, take these opportunities to reflect on your effectiveness, your feelings, and what you would do differently.

NOTES

_____

_____

_____

_____

_____

_____

_____

_____

_____

_____

_____

_____

_____

_____

_____

_____

_____

_____

_____

_____

_____

_____

_____

_____

_____

Chapter 11

THE 5Ws OF NEGOTIATING

Doc: *Dr. Bonnie, I retained an attorney just like you advised, and she did all of my negotiating for me.*

Dr. Bonnie: *I see. How was that received by your new practice?*

Doc: *Well, they didn't seem to like it, and now I am sensing some uneasiness from my new partners.*

Dr. Bonnie: *Yes, it's always best to negotiate on your own behalf, because you need to build ongoing relationships with your new partners, not your attorney.*

Welcome to your Discomfort Zone – Negotiations Know-How!

Welcome to your discomfort zone of contract negotiations. I know that might make us feel uncomfortable, but we've been in uncomfortable situations before and survived!

Dr. LaSalle Leffall, Jr. a highly revered general surgeon and physician educator at Howard University Hospital, encouraged all physicians under his tutelage to always maintain,

"Equanimity under duress."

Regardless of whether we are in the trauma bay, running a code in the intensive care unit, or managing a difficult delivery, we have learned how to tackle the uncertainty by being prepared and remaining as calm as possible. From studying to collecting relevant labs with hands-on experience empowers us to act in a patient care setting based on our knowledge and preparation, despite certain feelings of trepidation and anxiety. Quite simply, we have mastered this concept already.

We can now apply a similar data-driven approach to negotiating, and because of our training, we can do so successfully in spite of the uneasy feelings that negotiating may provoke.

This chapter will outline the core components of a negotiation strategy by focusing on the 5Ws of negotiating:

- o Who
- o What
- o When
- o Where
- o Why
- o and How

This is my attempt at simplifying the negotiation process, from one doctor to another doctor, in a way that makes this information digestible so that we can negotiate successfully in any situation. Then, in the next chapter, we will take our new understanding of these core components to build a customized negotiation strategy that will help us feel confident in any negotiating situation.

The 5 Ws of Negotiating

We will be discussing the nuts and bolts of negotiating from the perspective of looking at the five Ws: who, what, when, where, why, and how to negotiate.

Thinking about negotiations by examining the 5Ws reflects the method that I have used over the past several years, having mentored and coached hundreds of doctors through successful contract negotiations for employment, resignation, and leadership promotions.

Let's get started with "WHY" - Why are we negotiating in the first place?

One of the primary reasons that we are going to engage in negotiations is that we now KNOW that the contract that we are being offered is most often written in favor of the author of the contract, which we covered this concept extensively in Chapter 1.

Another classic negotiating concept is that we should expect (or least we should not be surprised) when the other party works to minimize their investment while expecting a maximal return. For example, we should expect that the first contract being offered may reflect the minimum amounts of compensation, leave, etc., in return for a maximum level of productivity and hours spent rendering patient care in exchange. Now, certainly this does not apply to every contract from every employer, but we must face the possibility of this being a more common reality for us. Thus, we must negotiate to ensure that our needs and wants are included in our employment agreement, as explained in Chapter 2.

The Compensation Gap

The reason we find disparities when it comes to compensation and benefits is that, unfortunately, as doctors, we have bought into the notion that we should not talk about money, compensation, and contracts. We have been taught not to share this information with each other throughout our medical education and training, because it was deemed immoral or unethical.

Certainly, nondisclosure and confidentiality terms exist within contracts that limit sharing of specific details and business practices. Yet, while you may not be allowed to discuss the particulars of how this organization works or functions, you can utilize your resources, references, and networks to learn about what is customary in that prospective work environment. In addition, negotiating for fair market value is the only way for us to close the compensation gap, which should be important to every doctor regardless of gender.

> ***Power Move #53** - We have to negotiate for our worth. Period!*

The "WHO" of Negotiating

An important point of clarification at the outset of negotiations is to understand with whom we are negotiating.

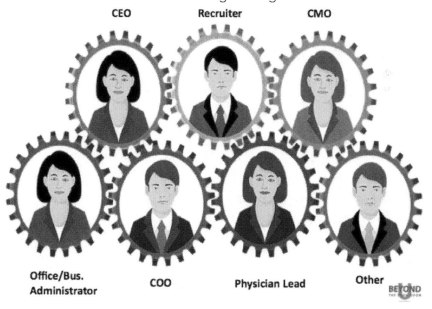

There are a number of professionals with whom you could possibly be negotiating the terms of your employment, including:

o   CEO – Chief Executive Officer – who may or may not be a doctor
o   CMO – Chief Medical Officer – who may be a doctor or nurse
o   Physician Lead – the doctor who would likely be your immediate supervisor
o   Recruiter/ Physician Liaison – the person assigned to communicate between you and the decision-maker(s) in the practice
o   Business Manager/Office Administrator – a person who is also likely to communicate between you and the decision-maker(s) in the practice

Part of your responsibility is to identify the role of the negotiator primarily so that you can ascertain whether this person:

o   has decision-making power
o   serves as the person communicating between you and the decision-maker

Negotiations with the decision-maker, such as the CEO or CMO, can sometimes be more expeditious because there is no middle person. Negotiating directly with a decision-maker allows us the opportunity to start building critical professional relationships early. It amplifies the new relationship that we are building because we want to always maintain an open line of communication with the decision-makers during negotiations and after we begin working in that environment.

> *Power Move #54 - Always build a relationship with the senior leaders in the practice or academic department, because having advocates in sponsors who support us in practice, in good times and in bad, is critical.*

Alternatively, negotiating with the middle person, such as a recruiter or business administrator, requires that we build a good relationship with this person so that they can accurately describe our needs/wants to the actual decision-makers.

> **Red Flag:** This middle person may sometimes be a recruiter or physician liaison. Always remember that recruiters are salespeople, and the primary goal of a salesperson is to close the deal by having you sign the contract, many times in an expeditious fashion. It is important to not succumb to any external pressure to sign a contract in 5, 10, or 20 days. Rather, having 30-60 days to do our due diligence by reviewing the contract ourselves and with our team of trusted advisors is customary and standard. Certainly, this scenario does not apply to everyone, but it is important to be aware.

Power Move #55 - *Do not sign any contract without adequate time to review it yourself and with your advisors.*

In addition, we can learn a lot by understanding the roles and relationships between the key people working for a prospective future employer. Through making key observations, we can learn a ton about the organization's:

o   Culture
o   Efficacy of the practice's leadership
o   Level of being doctor-supportive (or not)
o   Attention to detail
o   Communication styles and preferences

These are the types of observational assessments that you should be making consciously throughout the series of critical conversations that you will have during your negotiations, interviews, and second looks.

In the end, regardless of the role of the person that you are negotiating with, it is important to always be professional and respectful as you are building new relationships with everyone in a new environment. Remember, you will not have full knowledge of the existing relationships within the organization, so be sure to remain alert and non-disparaging throughout your negotiations.

Next, we want to talk about exactly "WHAT" you are negotiating.

"WHAT" is being negotiated

Priority #1 – Our Needs and Wants

Because your contract is the single most important document that dictates both your professional and personal life, we want to make sure that it comprehensively represents our needs (remember non-negotiable, i.e., dealbreakers). Also, as previously stated, negotiating at least some of your wants integrated into the contract is ideal, as well.

However, the doctor (that's YOU) has to be crystal clear about what will allow this negotiation to end in a win-win situation. No one can do this reflective, introspective work for you. I highly recommend that these exercises found in chapter 2 be completed PRIOR to engaging in negotiations. Consider having conversations with your accountability partner, family, and trusted advisors to think about the actual professional and personal aspects of your life that you need woven into this contract.

Thus, having your needs, priorities, protections, and options reflected in the contract are the components that make a contract a "good contract" for you and your family. This is your #1 priority, and we will talk about HOW to effectively negotiate these terms into your contract momentarily.

> *Power Move #56 - (worth repeating): Identifying our needs and wants prior to beginning negotiations increases the chances of our negotiations ending in a win-win for both parties.*

Priority #2 – Bi-directional Expectations

Your next priority in negotiations is understanding what is going to be expected from you in this position and what you can expect from the employer. Specific attention and clarification should be paid to the duties and responsibilities, including clinical, research, administrative, teaching, and perhaps leadership duties (which may include meeting attendance). Make sure that you have a full understanding of what is being proposed and be prepared to negotiate where you deem necessary.

For example, if you are negotiating on the subject of on-call duties, understand whether pay for call is standard within your region for your specialty and type of practice. If pay for call is, in fact, customary, but there is no compensation for call indicated in the contract, then this is a point that you will need to negotiate by researching the fair market value for payment in that region and for your specialty.

> *Power Move #57 - Negotiating from a data-driven and supported perspective improves our confidence levels and makes us more effective negotiators.*

Priority #3 – Top 5 Most Important Contract Terms

Hopefully, we are in agreement that the most important point of negotiation is NOT salary alone.

Instead, we want to remember the Top 5 contract terms that all doctors need to negotiate, including:

- o Term and termination
- o Non-compete clause
- o Malpractice Insurance
- o Fringe Benefits
- o Intellectual Property

Please review and have crucial conversations around these top 5 terms first, then move on to negotiating your total compensation package. Why? Because these are the key terms that confer the professional and personal protections that we need in order to live the fulfilled life that we deserve.

The "WHEN" of the Negotiations Process

As we move into the next steps, your strategy around when, where, and ultimately how to negotiate, let's quickly review a 10-Step Comprehensive Timeline and process for finding, negotiating, and securing a new position.

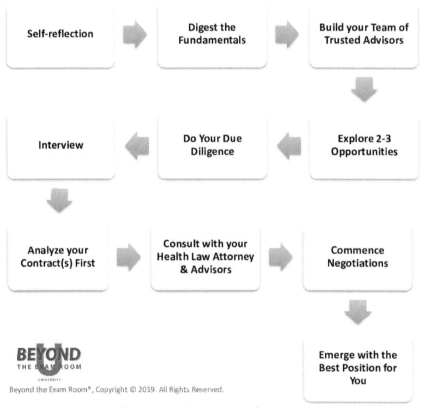

Figure 20 – The 10-Step Contracts and Negotiating Process

For Educational Purposes Only. Not Intended as Legal Advice.

We have spent the lion's share of this book demystifying the steps involved in the process of analyzing and negotiating an employment contract, a process that should ideally start 12-18 months prior to the date that you wish to start your new position. These steps consist of:

1. Engaging in self-reflection to discover our "Needs and Wants"
2. Learning and digesting the fundamentals of contracts, negotiations, finances, etc.
3. Building our "Team of Trusted Advisors"
4. Exploring 2-3 potential job opportunities by submitting a letter of interest and CV
5. Doing our due diligence in researching more about these opportunities
6. Interviewing with each practice
7. If there is a potential fit and a job offer is extended, then analyzing the letter of intent or contract(s) first,
8. Conferring and reviewing the letter of intent or contract with our Team of Trusted Advisors
9. Engaging in a series of crucial conversations during the formal negotiations period
10. After comparing our options, making an informed decision on the best position

To answer the question regarding when we start negotiating, these are the steps that lead up to and follow the formal negotiations process, seen here at Step 9. Once you have interviewed with a practice and a formal offer is extended, then the contracts and negotiations process has commenced. The first document you receive may be a letter of intent, or it may be the employment contract itself.

However, please know that you are being evaluated and interviewed from the moment that you make first contact with a practice and at every point in between. So, literally from the time you make your first inquiry with the practice about its available positions, you have already launched this entire process.

A Word of Caution about the Letter of Intent/Offer Letter/Term Sheet

Once you receive a letter of intent, consider yourself as having engaged affirmatively in the contracting process with this particular organization, even if the letter of intent states that it is nonbinding. By signing the letter of intent, you are giving this organization the green light that you want to move forward with the contract and negotiations process.

However, if you are not sure or if you need more time to review this letter of intent with your advisors, I would recommend that you do not sign the letter even if you have received a request to do so within a five-day period of receipt of the letter.

NOTE: Most organizations, if they are reasonable, are interested in getting the highest quality and caliber of doctor to come on board. Most doctor-supportive organizations and practices will understand a request for more time to do your due diligence.

If not, be willing to walk away and pursue your other 1-2 options.

"WHERE" do we negotiate?

Finally, we covered the best practice for where to negotiate in the previous chapter on the Top Negotiation Mistakes that Doctors Make.

I will reiterate, the goal is to negotiate face to face, if possible. If you're negotiating for a position long distance, then multiple face to face conversations are unlikely to happen. However, most negotiations should take place verbally over the phone rather than having the primary mode of communication take place via email or text.

Again, this is an exercise in relationship building, and you want to build this professional relationship in a way where you can pick up as many emotional and physical cues as possible, and the best way to do this is by speaking to the person.

Now, let's move into HOW to develop a negotiation strategy using all of these components.

CHAPTER SUMMARY

POWER MOVES

- o Who – Knowing with whom you are negotiating is a critical piece of preparing to negotiate effectively.
- o What – Your priorities of WHAT you are negotiating should include:
    - o Your needs and wants
    - o Expectations from both parties
    - o Top 5 contract terms
    - o Your total compensation package
    - o Additionally, knowing with whom you are negotiating is a critical piece of preparing to negotiate effectively.
- o When – Give yourself the gift of time, at least 12-18 months, when researching and ultimately negotiating for your first or next employed position.
- o Where – Make every attempt to negotiate person-to-person and avoid negotiations that take place only via email or text.

RED FLAGS

- o Any organization that pressures us into signing a contract within an expedited, e.g., five-day period of time may be indicating that they are not as doctor friendly as others.

NOTES

_____

_____

_____

_____

_____

_____

_____

_____

_____

_____

_____

_____

_____

_____

_____

_____

_____

_____

_____

_____

_____

_____

_____

_____

_____

For Educational Purposes Only. Not Intended as Legal Advice.

Chapter 12

BUILD YOUR NEGOTIATION KNOW-HOW STRATEGY

Doc: *Dr. Bonnie, you've convinced me that I need to negotiate, but I am terrified and I don't know how to do this.*

Dr. Bonnie: *No worries. Negotiating is a process that takes time, planning and preparation. Once you master how to build this strategy, you'll be able to apply it to other aspects of your life.*

In the world of business, negotiating is commonplace and expected. We know that this is the opposite for us as doctors. Negotiations are definitely foreign territory, so here are some practical tips that any doctor can use when preparing to negotiate. Honestly, these are tips that anyone can use in preparation for any negotiation that we are facing.

In this chapter, we will explore:

- o   The Negotiation Know-How Prep Process
- o   Building your negotiation strategy using the Sandwich Approach
- o   Winning Negotiation Tips

Everyday Negotiations

One last reminder to reinforce our ability to negotiate successfully includes reviewing the following list which reveals the plethora of opportunities we encounter regularly to engage in critical conversations and negotiations.

When participating in professional and development activities with:

- o   Healthcare teams
- o   Administrators
- o   Committees
- o   Board of Directors
- o   Patients and their families

In our personal lives and development:

- o   Spouse
- o   Partners
- o   Our Family
- o   Friends & associates

Unfortunately, our unwillingness to have these critical conversations fails us in many ways, and can result in:

- o Poor communication
- o Conflict resolution or not
- o Problem-solving or not
- o Understanding/confusion
- o Lack of Team building
- o Mistrust

The point here is that when we master the art of negotiating and having critical conversations that most of us would rather avoid, the positive impact will pervade our professional and personal lives, ultimately improving our interactions with others.

Just as we study for months to take a board exam, we must also take ample time (weeks) to do our due diligence and build a strategy as we prepare to negotiate during a critical conversation that may last an hour.

BEFORE THE NEGOTIATIONS – Power Moves Negotiation Prep Process

So, let's delve into "HOW" to negotiate successfully every time by taking these steps to prepare for your negotiations FIRST!

Before entering into any negotiation situation, you must prepare ahead of time. You will need sufficient time to implement the following steps to engage the other party with positive energy and affirming thoughts, to handle a potentially challenging situation with poise, preparation, and maturity.

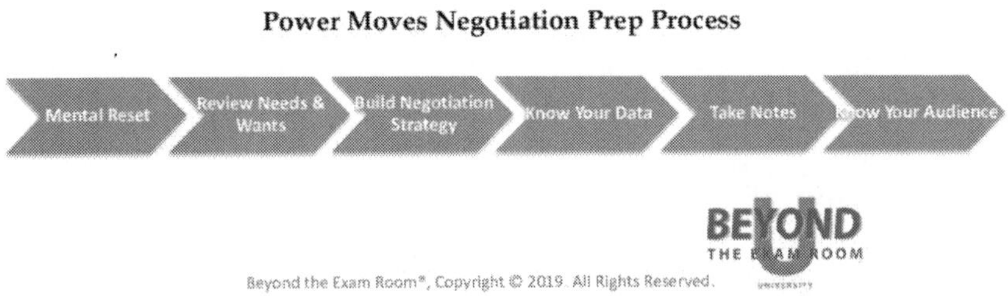

Power Moves Negotiation Prep Process

Mental Reset → Review Needs & Wants → Build Negotiation Strategy → Know Your Data → Take Notes → Know Your Audience

BEYOND
THE EXAM ROOM
UNIVERSITY

Figure 21 – Power Moves Negotiation Prep Process

We will begin with some of the mental and emotional steps that you should take before entering your negotiation:

Step 1 – Reset your mind. Affirm mentally that the primary goals of this critical conversation are to communicate effectively and to successfully exchange thoughts and ideas. Both of these goals require clear verbalization and active listening.

Because the idea of negotiating is so daunting, we must decide ahead of time that this is a communication exercise that we are capable of having successfully. Maintaining a positive mindset will pay off by setting a positive tone for your negotiation, and it's critical that you take time to do so perhaps 15 minutes before walking into that negotiation meeting or picking up the phone to call.

Also, I often avail myself to my doctor-clients if they need a pep talk for reassurance just prior to negotiating. So, phone a friend, which can work to settle and refocus your thoughts on the task at hand. We can do this!

I read the following in an advertisement in an airline's magazine,

"You don't get what you deserve. You get what you negotiate for!"

We have to remember this when we are negotiating our employment contracts.

> *Power Move #58* - *If we do not ask, we will not receive.*

Step 2 – Review your Needs and Wants. Review your Power Moves Needs and Wants Blueprint prior to your negotiations. You will need to review your specific wants and needs before entering into your critical conversation so that they will be fresh in your mind. Thinking about your needs and wants should also serve as a point of empowerment, because you have clarity about how the negotiations can end with a win-win from your perspective!

Step 3 - Organize your Negotiation Strategy. Develop your prioritized 3-point sandwich negotiation strategy ahead of time. This is where we apply the SIP to Success Strategy™ to negotiations. Proactively planning and practicing your talking points ahead of time is the secret to winning at negotiations.

1. After receiving your letter of intent or your contract, arrange to have a critical conversation with the prospective employer.
2. Prior to your meeting, meet with your coach or accountability partner to identify the 3 most important terms that you would like to discuss during your meeting.
3. These 3 most important terms must then be organized such that the most challenging contract term is discussed between two aspects of the contract that are relatively easier for both parties to discuss, hence the Sandwich reference.

Without this level of planning, your critical conversation, aka your negotiation, can feel very unnerving, disruptive, and unorganized likely yielding suboptimal
outcomes.

Step 4 - Know your data. Understanding the key data points and metrics surrounding your employment position is critical.
These data points include:

o   External metrics such as the average starting salary for your specialty in your region
o   The average number of RVUs generated by doctors in your stage of practice specialty and region
o   The average amount of revenue that positions in your specialty generate for the hospital on an annual basis
o   Specialty and state-specific terms that are customary for your specialty, such as the non-compete clause liability terms
o   Your first time cleaning claims submission rate versus denials, if you are a practicing doctor transitioning into another practice

Step 5 - Take Notes. Be prepared to take notes during the critical conversation, and let the other party know that you are doing so intentionally. As a matter of fact, taking notes during a critical conversation will serve three purposes:

- o Note-taking will allow you to capture the details of a relatively stressful conversation that you will most certainly miss if you do not document, primarily because you are stressed.
- o Note-taking also allows for a physical outlet during the critical conversation. If you become too nervous, you can always take a moment to pause and look down at your notes, especially to help you recall your speaking points. Please inform your interviewer that you are taking notes so that you can capture the details of the conversation and that you are not being rude or inattentive.
- o Taking notes also conveys a sense of being detail-oriented because you give the appearance of someone who does not want to miss the important aspects of the conversation. In doing so, you're making a great impression on the interviewer. You also have notes to reference during your follow-up email to the interviewer that recap your critical conversation.

> Red Flag - Do not take notes on your digital device. Handwrite your notes in a small journal or notebook. Using a digital device during an interview is the death wish since most interviewers may or may not be convinced that you were taking notes versus being on Instagram.

Step 6 - Know your audience. Finally, you must also know the core values of the potential employer or corporation that you may be working for, which can usually be found on the practice's website. This will inform you as to whether your goals and values are aligned with the practice, and it will serve as a good discussion point during your interview and/or in subsequent conversations. Do not forget to familiarize yourself with the names, titles, and roles of those with whom you will be interviewing.

As you can see from these 6 negotiation prep steps, negotiations are not to be entered into lightly or without preparation. Now, when entering your critical conversation, you will feel more empowered, knowledgeable, and prepared to have this conversation. As the Girl Scouts of America motto goes, "Be prepared."

DURING THE NEGOTIATIONS – Use the Sandwich Approach

Now, we can aggregate all of the aforementioned information, resources, and processes into my recommended framework for negotiating via critical conversations.

After coaching several groups of doctors through their respective negotiations, I began to recognize a common approach, which proved to be useful in each of their situations.

The 4 Parts of a Critical Conversation during your Negotiations

There are four components of a critical conversation that should take place in the sequential order:

1. The Top Slice Bread – Express Gratitude
2. Condiments – Build a rapport, and find common ground
3. The Meat (or Tofu) – Discuss the core points of negotiation
   a. Open with a point that yields an "easy yes"
   b. Then discuss stickiest points, i.e., the points where agreement has not yet been achieved
   c. End with another "easy yes"
4. The Bottom Slice of Bread – End with gratitude

Structuring ANY type of critical conversation in this fashion gives us the best possible chance of having the negotiation end in terms that are favorable, even if we have to bend on some of our points of negotiation.

This is why just "winging" it or hoping that a negotiation conversation will go well is not recommended. Let's explore each of these steps of the Sandwich approach in more detail:

1) First, express appreciation! After extending a firm hello, set the tone for the conversation by expressing your appreciation for the opportunity to interview. A spirit of graciousness and gratitude will provide and infuse the room with positive energy and lets the interviewer know that you come in peace, despite this being a negotiation.

> **Example**: Good morning, Dr. Brown, thank you so much for taking the time to speak with me today. I'm greatly appreciative and excited about learning more about your organization and this department. I know with your busy schedule that it is challenging to take time out. Thank you in advance.

2) Secondly, build a rapport! Understand that your goal is to build a rapport with the interviewer, especially if this is someone with whom you'll be working in the future, i.e., the department chair, doctor colleague, or even a future administrator.

Key to building rapport and getting to know someone is being able to articulate who you are clearly and concisely. One way to do this is to make sure that you articulate your core values and how they align with those of the organization and leadership in your prospective position.

By building bridges early and strategically, you are asserting the win-win. You are letting the party know that you have something in common and that your ultimate goal is to be of benefit to the organization using a professional skill set, but also to create a winning situation for yourself and your family. Win-win is hard to debate, because everyone wants to win.

Affirming the win-win also asserts that you are open and willing to communicate, such that both parties leave the discussion as satisfied as possible. It really works to defuse any tension or negativity that may be inherent to the critical conversation, aka the negotiation process.

Sample Language: I understand from your website that one of the core values of this organization is putting the doctors' needs first, because you understand that when doctors win, everyone wins. This aligns with one of my core values actually, which is teamwork. I believe that doctors, especially when we are supported and work together, can achieve maximum quality outcomes for our patients, which is the ultimate goal here. I was very happy to hear/read about your doctor-first culture, because I think we can achieve a win-win here today during this conversation.

3) Next, implement your 3-point sandwich negotiation strategy. The key points that you would like to negotiate from your contract should be thoroughly assessed prior to entering the room because you want to prioritize your discussion points during this critical conversation.

Point 1 - Your first discussion point should be a question or point of discussion where you are likely to get an easy "yes," an affirmative response to your request.

Point 2 - Your second discussion point should include your stickiest point of discussion. This discussion may focus on one or more of the top 5 contract terms or around compensation. Strategically, because you are sandwiching the stickier discussion on points you have already obtained yeses on, it actually drives your sense of confidence during this conversation. It is also affirming for potential employers that you and this person can, in fact, work together.

Point 3 - Your final point should also be a relatively easy "yes" for the both of you. Again, continue the positive energy and strong congenial momentum during this critical conversation. Your job at this time is not only to close the critical conversation with the win, but it is also to make sure that all of your true non-negotiables have been addressed.

4) Lastly, wrap it up nicely. After speaking about all of your prioritized discussion points and having done so in a successful fashion, you can now close the conversation by reiterating your appreciation and assertion that you have met the win-win criteria that you created at the beginning of the conversation. By reiterating steps one and two of your critical conversations, you have demonstrated your ability to be an effective communicator and to be a potentially excellent team member, coworker, and leader as a future employee of this organization.

AFTER THE NEGOTIATIONS – The Future is in the Follow-up!

After all, the future is in the follow-up, as one of my mentors told me years ago.

As previously stated, follow all verbal conversations during negotiations with an email, which is date and time-stamped to recant the details of the conversation, along with the points of consensus that were reached. Refer back to Chapter 3 to review the components of your email follow-up in an effort to be intentional with our documentation.

NEGOTIATION STRATEGIES FOR DOCTORS

Finally, let's end this chapter with some general negotiating tips that we should all review prior to negotiating our employment agreement:

1. One of the golden rules when it comes to contracts is that all contracts can be negotiated, utilizing similar and dissimilar strategies, depending on your position of strength or weakness.
2. First, you must understand that contracts usually benefit the writer of the contract, so it is up to you to dissect and negotiate the terms of the contract so that it will benefit you, as well.
3. Next, when it comes to negotiating, everything is negotiable once you understand what is negotiable.

4. The most important negotiation point is NOT salary alone.
5. Most practices will make an offer that is close to the national average, but we must do our compensation research first.
6. Be very careful obtaining outside advice on "reasonable salaries." Research the Fair Market Value for compensation in your specialty, region, and years in practice.
7. Speak to people who have recently SIGNED contracts in the type of practice that you are considering joining. Be assertive in collecting information from people who have recently transitioned successfully (or not).
8. Compare apples to apples, not apples to oranges.
   a. For example, consider the source when taking advice from private practitioners when you're looking at academic practices
   b. Similarly, consider the source when receiving advice from academicians when you're looking at private practices
9. Again, negotiate everything that CAN be negotiated. Finally, approach contract negotiations seriously, objectively, and with appropriate counsel.
10. Never let them see you sweat applies in that you should avoid emotional or hasty decisions when it comes to signing any contract.

CHAPTER SUMMARY

POWER MOVES

- o Negotiate on your own behalf after developing and practicing your negotiation strategy before you start to negotiate or terminate.
- o Take time to complete your 6-step Power Moves Negotiation Prep Process.
- o Build your Sandwich Approach to your negotiation strategy.

TAKE-HOME POINTS

- o Each of us will have a different negotiation strategy based on our unique needs (non-negotiables) and wants (negotiables).

RED FLAGS

- o Never have ANY critical or negotiation without taking the time to properly prepare.

HOMEWORK

- o Build your Sandwich Approach to your negotiation strategy using the Power Moves Negotiation Strategy Template.

NOTES

_____

_____

_____

_____

_____

Chapter 13

RENEGOTIATIONS AND RESIGNATIONS

Doc: *Dr. Bonnie, I quit my job earlier this morning.*

Dr. Bonnie: *Ummmm...you need to send me your contract immediately.*

Doc: *Why?*

Dr. Bonnie: *Well, just because you quit doesn't mean that everything is okay. Resigning also requires some important negotiating in order to protect yourself financially, your credentials and your license. We've got some work to do.*

I love the fact that negotiations are not limited to those who are transitioning into a practice, but also to those who are renewing their contracts, and those transitioning out of a practice.

> *Power Move #59 - In most situations, you can negotiate your transition into, through, and out of a practice using the Power Moves Negotiation Strategy from Chapter 12.*

LET'S RENEGOTIATE

However, I wanted to take a moment to address the #1 mistake that doctors make when renegotiating employment contracts.

Top Renegotiating Mistake - We fail to negotiate the renewal of our contract in a timely fashion, if at all.

While we have maximum leverage before we sign our contract, there is a window of time where you can leverage your expertise and productivity. This is your renewal period, during which you can renegotiate your contract.

Essential to your contract renegotiation is to first and foremost identify the time frame in which we can renegotiate our contracts.

Step 1 - Start by identifying the:

> o termination date of your contract
> o the number of days in which each party has to give notification of renewal or non-renewal, usually 90 or 120 days prior to the termination date

Step 2 - Count backward on the calendar to the date that is 90 or 120 days prior to the contract's end date, and this 90-120 day period of time is your renewal period. This is the critical time frame during which you can review terms in the contract that you would like to have renegotiated.

Step 3 – Identify the person within the practice likely your supervisor or the person with whom you negotiated your original contract with and request a meeting to discuss the renewal terms of your contract.

Terms that are most commonly renegotiated are:

- o Compensation
- o Productivity or other clinical benchmarks
- o On-call duties and compensation for call
- o Time commitments
- o Location of clinical duties
- o Teaching, Administrative, or Research duties

Any number of scenarios could prompt a doctor to renegotiate their contracts. Here are a few examples. Perhaps you have:

- o surpassed your productivity benchmarks for the past two years of your contract, then you could negotiate for a higher productivity bonus
- o submitted clean claims for 95% of your patients giving you a 95% clean claims submission rate, then you could negotiate for a higher percentile of RVU compensation
- o been working in a salaried position for 5 or 7 years without a pay raise, then negotiating for a cost of living raise is within reason

It is during this renewal period that we should proactively renegotiate the terms of the contract that apply to your situation.

> **Power Move #60** - Remember that everything is negotiable that is negotiable and that you get 0% of what you don't ask for.

BEFORE YOU RESIGN

Resigning from any position is another critical area where we must be strategic, intentional, and proactive.

Strategic planning is necessary to avoid undue professional, legal, financial, and emotional stress in an already stressful period of transition.

> **Power Move #61** - *Build a transition/exit strategy BEFORE you resign from your position.*

In my experience, the top mistake that doctors make when transitioning out of a practice is resigning without a plan. When they do so, it jeopardizes us in ways that are known and unknown to us. Certainly, there are urgent situations that require immediate transitions, yet even in those situations, if we can secure our professional and financial lives, let's do it by being strategic.

Because resigning from a position is ideally a relationship and career preserving negotiation, your resignation strategy will require:

1. Examining one's contract for the effects of termination
2. A series of critical conversations with the practice's decision-makers
3. Documentation of all communications during this period
4. Conferring with our team of trusted advisors, i.e., our attorney, financial advisor, and accountant
5. An analysis of the 14 points of financial vulnerability that doctors potentially face when transitioning out of a practice
6. Developing a projected transition budget to prevent destabilizing our lives
7. Ensuring that patient safety is not compromised
8. Signing of a separation agreement, in some situations, which may include a:
   a. non-disparagement clause
   b. severance pay
   c. communication guidelines for future credentialing inquiries, etc.

By building your transition/exit strategy based on the analysis and integration of all of the above, you can proceed with your transition using a data-driven, informed decision-making process.

I have received many phone calls from doctors who tell me, "I just quit my job!" Again, for all of the above reasons, we should not "just" quit. Think about it. Transitioning into this job required weeks of negotiating and a 20-page contract to secure the position. It will certainly take more than a one-paragraph email sent in haste to get us out of that position safely.

Because this process of transitioning out of a practice is indeed detailed and a bit beyond the scope of this book, I would like to invite all doctors to review my eBook entitled, *Before You Resign – The Doctor's Guide to Transitioning Smarter, Not Harder.*

CHAPTER SUMMARY

POWER MOVES

- o Negotiate your transition not just into a practice, but also during and when transitioning out of a practice situation.
- o SIP to Success when renegotiating and resigning.
- o Remember that everything is negotiable that is negotiable and that you get 0% of what you don't ask for.

TAKE-HOME POINTS

- o Devise a transition/exit strategy in conjunction with your team of advisors
- o Critical conversations regarding renegotiating your contract or resigning should take place person to person to be followed by email documentation of all details and the agreements reached.

RED FLAGS

- o Be careful not to be in breach of your contract by resigning in a way that jeopardizes:
- o patient care
- o your medical license
- o future credentialing
- o professional relationships

HOMEWORK

- o Identify the renewal date and your renewal period during which you will renegotiate your contract.

NOTES

_____

_____

Section 4

THE APPENDICES

Find clarity, get organized, and get paid!

THE APPENDICES

Appendix A – Playbook of Power Moves

Appendix B – The 10 - Step Contracts and Negotiating Process

Appendix C – Power Moves Points of Negotiation

Appendix D- Master Organization List of Documents for Trainees

Appendix E - Master Organization List of Documents for Practicing Physicians

Appendix F - Power Moves Anatomy of a Contract (Extended Version)

Appendix G - RISC Analysis™ Template

Appendix H - Power Moves Compensation Package

Appendix I – Power Moves Intellectual Property "Carve Out" List

Appendix A - Playbook of Power Moves

Power Move #1	ALWAYS REMEMBER that contracts are written in favor of the AUTHOR of the contract!
Power Move #2	Give yourself the gift of time during your job search!
Power Move #3	We must do our due diligence!
Power Move #4	SIP To SuccessTM Theory: S= Be Strategic I = Intentional Documentation P = Proactive Communication
Power Move #5	Forget Work-Life Balance. Consider Work-Life Integration!
Power Move #6	Doctors, we must know our needs and our wants, because WE matter!
Power Move #7	It is always our responsibility to advocate for ourselves by asking and negotiating for what WE need and want.
Power Move #8	All professionals need a coach. We are the star player on our own team, so let's build our team of expert advisors to help us navigate to the finish line, end zone or to the 18th hole, effectively and efficiently.
Power Move #9	Just as we do not base our research conclusions based on data collected from a sample size with an n =1, we have to check multiple references for each advisor, including those from other professionals and from other doctor-clients.
Power Move #10	Meet with your Trusted Advisors frequently, e.g. quarterly to semi-annually. Once you articulate your desire to meet routinely, your Trusted Advisor should be proactively working to engage you per your desire.
Power Move #11	Consult your Trusted Advisors when making ALL career, leadership, business, practice management, legal, and financial decisions.
Power Move #12	When reviewing contracts, allow time for each of your trusted advisors to review the agreement from their perspective, which gives you a comprehensive analysis of the potential opportunity.
Power Move #13	We are no longer going to make six-figure decisions in five days.
Power Move #14	Let's learn how to analyze our contracts, so that we can confer with our health law attorney, financial advisor and accountant as an informed client, so that we can develop an informed and strategic approach to our contract negotiations.

For Educational Purposes Only. Not Intended as Legal Advice.

Appendix A - Playbook of Power Moves (Cont.)

Power Move #15	Before you begin reading any contract, review the entire document to assess the different components of the contract, i.e., the face, the body, and the appendices/addendums.
Power Move #16	Verify that all pages included are in sequential order and that no pages are missing from the document, both before and after you sign.
Power Move #17	In order to build this new and critically important skill set, I recommend that every doctor read or earnestly attempt to read their own contract first, in preparation for discussing the contract with our health law attorney and our other trusted advisors.
Power Move #18	Analyzing a contract comes after reflecting on your needs and wants from Chapter 2.
Power Move #19	The process of negotiating our employment contract is an exercise in relationship-building. Therefore, the goal is to reach terms of mutual agreement, especially in the terms that represent your needs, aka your non-negotiables, while being communicative and collegial vs. being demanding and inflexible.
Power Move #20	If it's not in black and white → it doesn't count, and it does not have to be enforced.
Power Move #21	Following every negotiation conversation, always follow-up by sending the other party an email that is date and time stamped with which documents were reviewed and what was agreed upon in the conversation.
Power Move #22	Circle, highlight, or underline any vague term within the contract so that you can discuss it with your attorney before addressing it in your negotiations. This will expedite your discussion with your attorney and will empower you to be an informed client in working with them.
Power Move #23	Do your due diligence on the fair market value for compensation norms for your specialty, in your specific region and practice type. Don't forget to work your network of colleagues who have recently transitioned into the workforce.
Power Move #24	ALWAYS keep your own documentation on the numbers, diagnoses, and procedures. (After all, we documented our patients and cases in residency, so let's just keep it going.)
Power Move #25	Make sure you understand the buy-in calculation and/or the additional partnership eligibility requirements at the time that you sign the first employment agreement with the private practice.

For Educational Purposes Only. Not Intended as Legal Advice.

Appendix A - Playbook of Power Moves (Cont.)

Power Move #26	Ask as many questions as possible to assess the culture, fit, financial management, strategy, and plans, i.e., mergers, acquisitions, departures, or purchases, BEFORE signing on as a partner.
Power Move #27	As part of your due diligence, have your tax accountant, in addition to your health law attorney and your financial advisor, review your contract BEFORE signing on the dotted line.
Power Move #28	Review the terms of your insurance policies with your insurance broker, who may be your financial advisor, on an annual basis, or when major life events/transitions happen in your life.
Power Move #29	It is up to you to obtain copies of your own insurance policies and keep them in a secure digital file, as well as a hard copy, which should be kept in a fire-proof, waterproof safe. (See Appendix C & D for my Master Organization List of Documents that every doctor must have at their fingertips.)
Power Move #30	Take caution and time to do your due diligence when it comes to signing any contract.
Power Move #31	We do NOT make six-figure decisions in a five-day period of time!
Power Move #32	Always review these Top 5 Contract Terms in every contract: • Term and Termination • Non-compete Clause • Malpractice Insurance • Intellectual Property/ Outside Revenue Generation • Fringe Benefits
Power Move #33	If you are resigning, i.e., terminating your contract, I HIGHLY recommend that you resign in person FIRST, then submit a written letter of resignation NEXT. This direct person to person approach, followed by written documentation, will hopefully help to mitigate any potential negative consequences of your resignation.
Power Move #34	If the employer is terminating you without cause, then a point of negotiation before you even sign the initial contract is to assert that if the employer terminates your contract, then the employer: Nullifies the non-compete clause; Covers the cost of your tail policy, if applicable.
Power Move #35	While non-competes are usually not negotiated out of doctor employment contracts, the radius, duration, and medical services prohibited can usually be negotiated into terms that are agreeable to both parties by providing valid professional and/or personal reasons.
Power Move #36	Be aware that all contract language is not this clear. Take the time to clarify whether you are an employee or an independent contractor for yourself.

For Educational Purposes Only. Not Intended as Legal Advice.

Power Move #37	If you have any current or potential projects in development that are eligible to be patented, trademarked, for copyright with the potential for monetization, please develop your own list of intellectual property and proprietary works for submission as a "carve out."
Power Move #38	The signatures, titles, and dates of the signatures are required from both parties. Please note, if you are signing an agreement as an independent contractor who has his or her own corporate entity, such as an LLC, you should sign as a representative of your company, and not as an individual. Please work with your accountant to determine which corporate entity is best for you BEFORE signing any document.
Power Move #39	Calculate the total value of your compensation package, which is not just the salary amount in your paycheck.
Power Move #40	Be sure to review each aspect of your compensation with your accountant, financial advisor, and attorney in order to understand the tax implications, budgetary impacts, and legalities of your compensation package.
Power Move #41	Negotiate to obtain three quotes for the costs of your relocation and agree to accept the middle quote.
Power Move #42	All doctors should do their own coding! Take a coding course on an annual basis to understand medical coding and billing for your specialty, especially if you are in your first 3 years of practice.
Power Move #43	Maximize & DOCUMENT your productivity during your foundational years even while you are on a guaranteed salary!
Power Move #44	Intentionally document your productivity, i.e., the number, ICD-10, CPT codes for every patient that you see in every clinical setting (see the sample Productivity Tracker in Appendix E)
Power Move #45	Proactively communicate with administrators to review and verify the documentation of your productivity and the accurate calculation of your RVU calculations.
Power Move #46	Strategically work within your practice to ensure that your productivity is maximized.
Power Move #47	Strategically work with your financial advisor to develop a budget that can provide financial security in the event that your productivity and hence your compensation varies.
Power Move #48	I am changing my mindset around negotiating. I can do this!

For Educational Purposes Only. Not Intended as Legal Advice.

Appendix A - Playbook of Power Moves (Cont.)

Power Move #49	Consult our advisors → Collect our data → Build a Negotiation Strategy → Practice → Negotiate → Win!
Power Move #50	Remember that negotiating is part of a relationship-building process. So start building this relationship by negotiating for yourself and do so face to face, or at least person to person.
Power Move #51	Be intentional about documenting your critical conversations during negotiations (and in practice for that matter) by sending a follow-up email recap to the person with whom you are negotiating. This provides a date and time stamp along with a written record of what was covered and agreed/disagreed on during the conversation, which may be helpful for future reference.
Power Move #52	Consult our advisors → Collect our data → Build a Negotiation Strategy→ Practice → Negotiate → Win!
Power Move #53	We have to negotiate for our worth. Period!
Power Move #54	Always build a relationship with the senior leaders in the practice or academic department, because having advocates in sponsors who support us in practice, in good times and in bad, is critical.
Power Move #55	Do not sign any contract without adequate time to review it yourself and with your advisors.
Power Move #56	(worth repeating): Identifying our needs and wants prior to beginning negotiations increases the chances of our negotiations ending in a win-win for both parties.
Power Move #57	Negotiating from a data-driven and supported perspective improves our confidence levels and makes us more effective negotiators.
Power Move #58	If we do not ask, we will not receive.
Power Move #59	In most situations, you can negotiate your transition into, through, and out of a practice using the Power Moves Negotiation Strategy from Chapter 12.
Power Move #60	Remember that everything is negotiable that is negotiable and that you get 0% of what you don't ask for.
Power Move #61	Build a transition/exit strategy BEFORE you resign from your position.

Appendix B
The 10-Step Contracts and Negotiating Process – The Big Picture

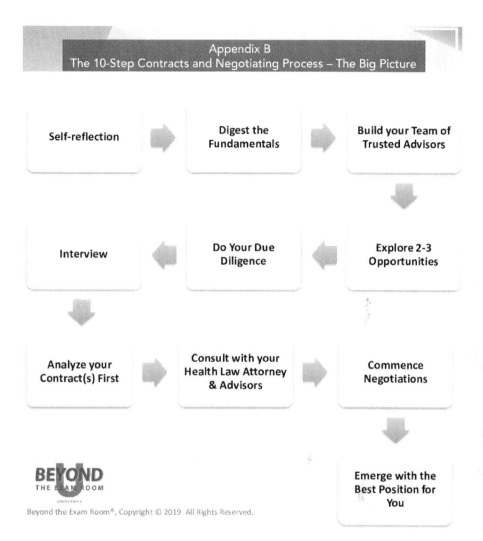

Self-reflection → Digest the Fundamentals → Build your Team of Trusted Advisors

Interview ← Do Your Due Diligence ← Explore 2-3 Opportunities

Analyze your Contract(s) First → Consult with your Health Law Attorney & Advisors → Commence Negotiations

Emerge with the Best Position for You

For Educational Purposes Only. Not Intended as Legal Advice.

Power Moves Sample Points of Negotiation

Time Commitment

- o Non-monetary items that affect your work and quality of life
  - o Duty hours in an outpatient setting
  - o Weekend or overnight responsibilities
  - o Schedule changes only with your consent
- o Shift work – primarily for independent contractors working on an hourly basis
  - o Understand the overtime trigger
- o Time and budget for community outreach

Life Accommodations

- o Additional Leave - PTO; Family leave +/- pd

Duties and Responsibilities

- o Administrative, teaching, clinical vs. research
- o Supervision of mid-levels & pay for supervision
- o On-call duties - pay for call, number and location of calls

Protections

- o Non-compete - radius, duration, primary practice designation
- o Intellectual Property

Partnership

- o Buy-ins, buy-outs, stock options, and the structure of each of these items

Academia

Request and negotiate for the funding sources (e.g. Grants, Departmental funds) for:
- o   Administrative duties
- o   Teaching duties
- o   Dedicated research time (if applicable)
- o   Clinical duties
- o   Leadership positions

Leadership Position
- o   Percentage of time (FTE) allocated to the leadership role
- o   Consider not just your individual but consider the needs of the entire department, division or office
  - o   Administrative support, CME time and/or resources for yourself and staff, Executive coaching, Analytic/statistical support

Productivity
- o   Bimonthly or Quarterly Productivity Reviews with Administration to verify productivity:
  - o   RVUs,
  - o   Collections
  - o   Overhead allocations
  - o   Pay allocations

Commuter Issues
- o   Commuter pay – consider when traveling to alternate clinical sites that may be an hour away from the main hospital
- o   Limits on travel distance AND time to and from satellite sites
- o   Negotiate for "Indemnification" which means to hold another party harmless. In this situation where a doctor may be commuting for work, negotiate to have the hospital indemnify you as an employee, e.g. means if you get in an accident or injure someone while driving between work sites i.e. Between hospital to hospital or hospital to clinic etc. the victim can only sue your hospital/company and not you personally.

Appendix D - Master Organization List of Documents for Trainees

PROFESSIONAL FILES

_____ Employment Contract
_____ LICENSES
_____ All state licenses with numbers and dates of issue/resignation
_____ DEA
_____ BOARD SCORES/RESULTS
_____ USMLE I, II, III
_____ Specialty Boards
_____ Medical School Diploma
_____ Residency Certificate
_____ National Board or equivalent
_____ College and medical school transcripts
_____ Fellowship Certificate
_____ Past 7 years of Business Tax Returns
_____ Loan Applications
_____ Financial Records

FOR EACH INSTITUTION YOU WORKED AT:

_____ Address and phone number
_____ Dates you received credentialing and dates you left
_____ Name, phone number of contact to verify your position
_____ Name, phone number of Department of Chairman, Program Director, Residency
_____ Coordinator
_____ Copy of Board Certification
_____ Copy of all documents regarding and lawsuit - NOTARIZED
_____ Copy of Annual CME's
_____ CV
_____ Keep record of CME courses attended
_____ Publications
_____ Presentations: # hours, # people present and audience
_____ Volunteer efforts
_____ Honors received

CONTACT LIST OF CONSULTANTS AND ACCOUNTS (if applicable):

_____ Banker
_____ Accountants
_____ Attorneys
_____ Financial Planner

PERSONAL FILES

- Notarized Copy of Birth Certificate
- Social Security Card
- Passport
- Immunization Records
- FRONT AND BACK COPIES OF:
- Driver's License
- Credit Cards
- Insurance Cards
- Will
- Revocable Living Trust
- INSURANCE POLICIES
- Health Plan
- Life
- Disability
- Property
- Automobile
- Umbrella
- Long-term Care
- Homeowner's Insurance
- Renter's Insurance
- TITLES OF OWNERSHIP
- Home
- Automobile
- Houses/apartments: list of addresses, phone numbers, dates
- Past 7 years Tax Returns

ADDITIONAL TIPS:

Photo files are important. Keeps photos on your phone of your drivers license, car insurance, car registration, and license plate, and passport.

On a secure cloud you can also upload credit card numbers, phone numbers for the cards (both national and international), travel insurance and passport information, so that you can access it anytime from any where.

Keep all of the above along with medical information in a sealed envelope with a friend who I can reach when traveling.

Appendix E - Master Organization List of Documents for Practicing Physicians

PROFESSIONAL FILES

_____	Employment Contract
_____	LICENSES
_____	All state licenses with numbers and dates of issue/resignation
_____	DEA
_____	BOARD SCORES/RESULTS
_____	USMLE I, II, III
_____	Specialty Boards
_____	Medical School Diploma
_____	Residency Certificate
_____	National Board or equivalent
_____	College and medical school transcripts
_____	Fellowship Certificate
_____	Past 7 years of Business Tax Returns
_____	Loan Applications
_____	Financial Records

FOR EACH INSTITUTION YOU WORKED AT:

_____	Address and phone number
_____	Dates you received credentialing and dates you left
_____	Name, phone number of contact to verify your position
_____	Name, phone number of Department of Chairman, Program Director, Residency Coordinator
_____	Copy of Board Certification
_____	Copy of all documents regarding and lawsuit - NOTARIZED
_____	Copy of Annual CME's
_____	CV
_____	Keep record of CME courses attended
_____	Publications
_____	Presentations: # hours, # people present and audience
_____	Volunteer efforts
_____	Honors received

CONTACT LIST OF CONSULTANTS AND ACCOUNTS (if applicable):

_____	Banker
_____	Accountants
_____	Attorneys
_____	Financial Planner

PERSONAL FILES

FRONT AND BACK COPIES OF:

- _____ Notarized Copy of Birth Certificate
- _____ Social Security Card
- _____ Passport
- _____ Immunization Records
- _____ Driver's License
- _____ Credit Cards
- _____ Insurance Cards
- _____ Will
- _____ Trust
- _____ Advanced Directives
- _____ Powers of Attorney

INSURANCE POLICIES

- _____ Health Plan
- _____ Life
- _____ Disability
- _____ Property
- _____ Automobile
- _____ Umbrella
- _____ Long-term Care
- _____ Homeowner's Insurance
- _____ Renter's Insurance

TITLES OF OWNERSHIP

- _____ Home
- _____ Automobile
- _____ Houses/apartments: list of addresses, phone numbers, dates
- _____ Past 7 years Tax Returns

ADDITIONAL TIPS:

Photo files are important. Keeps photos on your phone of your drivers license, car insurance, car registration, and license plate, and passport.

On a secure cloud you can also upload credit card numbers, phone numbers for the cards (both national and international), travel insurance and passport information, so that you can access it anytime from any where.

Keep all of the above along with medical information in a sealed envelope with a friend who I can reach when traveling.

Appendix F - Power Moves Anatomy of a Contract

Becoming familiar with a contract requires practice, and with repetition, a greater understanding and a decreased sense of anxiety can result, i.e. the more you give grand rounds, the more comfortable we become.

The goal of this chapter is to gain an understanding of the core components a contract, i.e. an agreement.

So, we will start building our understanding of a contract with dissecting and defining the key components of a contract with very literal anatomical references.

(At the risk of being too literal in this description of the parts of the contract, I will share a few comparisons to the human anatomy as a basis of reference. It may be a stretch, but indulge me. ☺)

ANATOMY OF THE PROCESS

Heart - As stated in Chapter 1, at the Heart of this entire contracts and negotiations is the physician, and the terms you need and want to have represented in the contract that represent:

- Your why – The core of who you are; your core values
- Your needs (non-negotiables, deal-breakers)
- Your wants (negotiables, nice to haves)
- Your perspective having integrated your work and your life

So once again, I beckon the gunners who are reading this book and have skipped Section 1, please take time to go back and review the entirety of that section so that you can do the pre-work necessary to achieve a win-win.

What if I don't?
I can't tell you how many physicians I have spoken over the years who have called me out of frustration with their positions, secondary to terminology in their contract that they did not understand. When I ask if they reviewed their contract, they profess, "Well, I had an attorney review my contract, but the contract did not meet my needs or requests."

Case in point, unless we take the time to review and share our needs/wants, our core values, and our priorities in the work-life integration model, then it is virtually impossible for any advisor to make sure that our interests are legally protected. Attorneys, financial advisors, bankers, etc. are not mind readers, nor should we expect them to be.

Brain (Central Nervous System) – After taking time to reflect on who we are, then its time for the Brain of the process to begin understanding the process of analyzing the contract and how to digest what we are reviewing in our pursuit of the Win-Win.

As discussed in Chapter X, we can use the RISC Analysis as a framework to analyze and review every term in the contract, prior to reviewing the contract with our health law attorney and other advisors.

- R – Reciprocity
- I – Important
- S – Specific
- C- Customary (Standard) Practices

This approach from a 30,000 foot view will hopefully help to decrease some of the angst that contract reviews can elicit from any individual, but especially as physician having usually been provided with minimal if any formal education in business, much less contract negotiations.

Now, let's compare the human anatomy and physiology to the most important terms of a physician's employment contract. The terms will be defined in detail in the subsequent chapter, but these analogies will help us build an overall context for understanding of THE MOST CRITICAL parts of the contract.

Integument ☐ Negotiations

Just as our outer appearance serves to communicate parts of who we are to the external environment, we can view the process of negotiating in the same light. Our skin, the with the largest surface area of any organ system in the body, serves to protect, serve as a sieve and filter of its own by absorbing Vitamin D, then repelling pollutants. In addition our skin and nails serve their own protective functions, as well. Further, how we choose to dress, our body language and external cues play a significant role in how we relate to others.

With this in mind, we should consider that negotiating is our outward communication of who we are, our intentions and expectations when we are considering a new position. We are vocalizing that we want to achieve a win-win while simultaneously exercising our contracts knowledge in order protect our best interest in the process. Therefore, when we do not negotiate out of fear or because we think that "they" won't like us deprives us of the opportunity to stand up for our own interests and to protect ourselves as the primary revenue generators healthcare.

In the end, we can elect how we choose to look and dress, just as we can choose to negotiate or not. I would submit that not negotiating could be likened to choosing not to wear clothing outside of the house leaving us susceptible and vulnerable. Assuming that most of us choose clothing, I hope that once you complete this book, that you tools and strategies you need to will feel educated and empowered to negotiate on behalf of yourself, your family and your patients.

Pulmonary System ☐ Term and Termination

Just as the ultimate and reciprocal gas exchange of oxygen and carbon dioxide occurs at the cellular level in our aveoli, your term and termination clauses in your employment agreement represents one of the top five most critical areas in your contract.

Why? Because the term of your contract represents the life expectancy of your contract and the termination clause is the opportunity for the employer and physician to reciprocally exchange and agree upon the plethora of circumstances under which your contract will end. The term and termination clauses represent the life and death of your contract.

Immune System ⮕ Malpractice Insurance & Fringe Benefits (Health, Life & Insurance Protections)

Because our immune confers critical, multi-system protections against both internal and external threats, compromise and disease, the insurance clauses in our contract serve the same protective purposes. Namely the malpractice insurance clause protects us from a professional perspective, while the life, disability, health insurance protections conferred as fringe benefits protect our #1 asset. We are our #1 asset, because we rely on our mental, physical and emotional capacities and capabilities to render healthcare, hence we must protect ourselves by paying close attention to these terms in our contract. For these reasons these two terms qualify for the top 5 most important contract terms, as well.

Sympathetic Nervous System ⮕ Covenant Not To Compete

Similarly, the non-compete clause, which is one of many Restrictive Covenants in an employment agreement, is a term written in to limit or eliminate the threat of competition that you, the physician, may pose once you leave a practice. Just as the Sympathetic Nervous System works to provide impose some barriers and limitations on the body, the non-compete does the same by limiting when and where you can practice in your specialty (or not) upon leaving a practice. Because of the gravity and breadth of impact on a physician's ability to practice in a given geographic region for a specified amount of time, this contract term certainly makes list of one of the top 5 most important terms in your contract.

Right Brain ⮕ Intellectual Property

Our ability to innovate, lead and problem solve creatively are the attributes that initially made us the ideal and most competitive candidate for medical school. As physicians engage in the art of medicine, research and the rendering of healthcare, we often identify voids and many times create solution-driven approaches to such issues. Our creative capacity certainly extends beyond medicine, also as our medical school and residency applications reflected.

My personal opinion: Even as practicing physicians, we should retain the rights to own our inventions, patents, copyrights, trademarks and licenses that result from our creative capacities. Our capacity to innovate, create, develop and drive change both within and outside of medicine should be protected.

With this said, physicians must review the specific intellectual property rights and the opportunities to generate outside revenue within our employment contract. It has been standard practice in academia that physicians yield their rights to own their own IP to the university or academic center. However, current trends in physician employment contracts from practices and locums agencies with no academic affiliations are limiting the IP ownership rights of employed physicians, even those who may be only working part-time.

Thus, the intellectual property clause rounds out the top 5 critically important terms in a physician's employment agreement.

Wait a minute! Compensation is not one of the top 5 most critical contract terms for physicians?

No, but it is the sixth most important contract term, and here is why.

Musculoskeletal System [] Compensation

Of course the orthopaedic surgeon in me would like to elevate the musculoskeletal system to the most important position in the level of importance in our contract, but in fact, I cannot. For we know that appendages are non-essential for sustaining life, but this system does power movement which is critical to maintaining life at optimal levels.

Similarly compensation powers the contract and our salary serves as the fuel in exchange for the excellent healthcare that we provide on a routine basis.

With that said, the musculoskeletal system and the power it provides cannot sustain the body's functions alone, not can this serve as our priority. Similarly, many a physician has only focused on the salary term of their contract, without giving due regard to the previously stated top 5 critical terms and have subsequently found themselves in dire situations.

While their six figure paychecks were being deposited, the limitations and negative impact of the sudden termination without cause, non-compete restrictions, lack of insurance protections when life happens or lost intellectual property revenue overshadowed the dollars in their bank accounts. Something to consider.

Gastrointestinal & Urologic Systems, specifically the GI Tract, Kidneys and Liver [] Your Team of Trusted Advisors

Just as our gastrointestinal and urologic Systems, specifically the GI tract, kidneys and liver, serve as primary sites of absorption of nutrients while filtering out waste, your team of trusted advisors should be viewed similarly. Once we have vetted and compiled our individual team of trusted advisors, we can then run critical contract, financial and personal information through each of them with the expectation that their expertise will help us filter out what we does not serve us during contract negotiations, transitions and major financial decisions. Hence, we partner with our trusted advisors to exchange ideas and implement strategies by communicating with them frequently and often.

Each advisor provides input through their respective lenses and in cooperation with one another to help us reach our overall professional and personal goals.

The face, which is the first section/paragraph in any contract, literally serves to list the following key definitions, which apply to the entirety of the remainder of the contract:

- The parties who are entering to the agreement, e.g. the Employer and Physician, the Hospital and the Contractor, the Lessee and Lessor.
- The names, addresses and corporate structure of the entities will be addressed in this first paragraph, as well.

- It is important to make sure that you are familiar with the references in this first section, because these are the references that will be used throughout the remainder of the contract.
- For example, the ABC Medical Center will be referred to as the "Employer," and Janice Doe, MD will be referred to as the "Employee." This sounds simple enough, but it can become confusing if references are made to multiple locations or multiple parties.
- Be sure to identify the addresses and/or locations of the medical center, which would also be defined in this initial paragraph, as many employers in particular have multiple office locations or satellites that may unknowingly apply to you.

The body of the contract will contain all of the main terms that govern the two parties entering into the agreement. There are standard terms that will be found in every contract, and these terms will be defined in the following chapter.

Though sometimes the names of these terms vary, standard contracts should include and address the following:

The 25 important subheadings are listed below, but what do these subheadings mean? We will deconstruct a contract and define each subheading before we deal with the actual contractual negotiations.

TERMINOLOGY

- Definitions
- Employment and Term
- Duties and Responsibilities
- Compensation
- Vacation/Personal time
- Fringe Benefits
- Expenses
- Moving Expenses
- Professional Liability
- Termination
- Covenant Not to Compete
- Non-disclosure
- Non-solicitation
- Reasonableness of Restrictions
- Ownership Opportunity
- Action by Authority with Legal Jurisdiction
- Representations of Physician
- Insurance
- Books, Records and Office Equipment
- Assignability
- Notices
- Severability
- Effect of termination
- Waiver
- Governing Law; Jurisdiction; Venue
- SIGNATURES

The exhibits, appendix (appendices) or addendum (addenda) could be compared to the appendages of the contract. Found at the end of the body of the contract following the signatures from both parties, these additional contract components address in further or customized detail one of the terms in the body of the contract.

Commonly, the appendix may contain details pertaining to the:

- Compensation package
- Benefits

Alternatively, the appendix will serve as the location of additional agreements that serve as supplements to the primary contract, such as:

- Promissory note (this is a loan agreement)
- Income guarantee (also a loan agreement)

ANATOMY OF A CONTRACT - CHAPTER SUMMARY

Key Business Tips

Take Home Points/Gold Standard/Best Practices

- Before you begin reading any contract, review the entire document to assess the different components of the contract, i.e. the face, the body and the appendices/addendums.
- Verify that all pages included are in sequential order and that no pages are missing from the document, both before and after you sign.

Red Flags

- Always, always, always read the appendices/addendums to the contract. Many vital details hide here.
- At the end of the contract process, in addition to obtaining signatures from both parties, insist on having both parties initial each page, along with any manual corrections that need to be made.

Appendix G - The RISC™ Analysis Framework

R - Reciprocal

I – Important (to me)

S - Specific

C - Customary

Appendix H - Comprehensive Compensation Package Components

Salary	Benefits	Leave
Base Pay	**Insurance Protections**	**Administrative**
Gross vs. Net	- Malpractice	CMEs +/- pd fees
- Guaranteed Salary	- Life	Personal
- Productivity-Based	- Disability	Sick Leave
- Quality-Based	- Health	Maternity/ Paternity
- Net-Revenue Based	- Dental	
	- Vision	**Other**
Variable Pay	- Long-Term Care	Dues, Licenses
- Signing Bonus		Relocation Exp
- Productivity Bonus	**Savings/Retirement**	Cell phone, Parking
- Loan Repayment	- 401k, 403b, Pension	Travel
- Forgivable Loan	- +/- matching funds	- Airfare
- Partnership Draws	- Health Savings Acct	- Auto
	- Thrift Savings Plan	

Appendix I - Power Moves Intellectual Property "Carve Out" List

Licenses, copyrights, patents, trademarks/service marks

Corporations, Partnerships or other businesses

Investments

Intellectual Property

Original Works - Type of content with Titles
- o Books (Hard Copy Digital)
  - o Fiction and non-fiction
  - o Coloring books
  - o Policies and procedures
    - Manuals, guides or workbooks
    - Photography, artwork
    - Music

Public Speaking - Type of content with Titles
- o Content
- o Associated Honoraria

Products

- o Medical Devices
- o Digital Products
  - o Software
  - o Apps
  - o Websites
  - o Blogs
  - o eBooks
  - o Online courses
  - o Webinars
  - o Social Media
  - o Podcasts
- o Merchandise
- o Cosmetics

Services

- o Coaching
- o Consulting
- o Education

For Educational Purposes Only. Not Intended as Legal Advice.

ABOUT THE AUTHOR

Dr. Bonnie Simpson Mason has committed the entirety of her career to educating and empowering her current and future physician colleagues. As a self-proclaimed innovator, void-filler and driver of solutions, Dr. Mason believes that with the right information, tools and resources that all students, residents and physicians can be successful, both professionally and personally.

Dr. Mason is also the Co-Founder/Chief Executive Officer of Beyond the Exam Room, where she has developed a comprehensive, CME-accredited business of medicine, career-development, leadership and financial curriculum that she has been delivering to young physicians in conjunction with physician colleagues and trusted advisors over the past 15 years.

Dr. Mason was the Founder and Executive Director of Nth Dimensions. Dr. Mason designed all aspects of execution and delivery of the Nth Dimensions physician pathway program and curriculum, to decrease disparities in the healthcare workplace by increasing the number of women and other underrepresented minorities in competitive specialties, including orthopedic surgery, radiology, dermatology, and ophthalmology. Her effectiveness over the past 15 years in diversity and inclusion was acknowledged by the American Academy of Orthopedic Surgery in 2015 with its Diversity Award.

Dr. Mason earned a Bachelor of Science degree in Chemistry from Howard University in Washington, DC, her Doctor of Medicine degree from Morehouse School of Medicine in Atlanta, Georgia, her general surgery internship at UCLA, completed her residency at Howard University Hospital in the Division of Orthopedic Surgery, where she was named Chief Resident of the Year. She served as a board-certified orthopedic surgeon and chief operating officer for her group practice in Washington, DC, and clinical assistant professor at Howard University; then as an adjunct associate professor at the University of Louisville in GME; and, is presently adjunct assistant professor at UTMB in Orthopedic Surgery and Rehabilitative Medicine.

Dr. Mason is most thankful for being a proud wife, mom of 2 future leaders and bestie to many.

INDEX

A
accountability partner, 27, 28, 32, 34, 44, 45, 47, 58, 59, 62, 64, 65, 250, 264
accountant, 72, 74, 91, 115, 117, 133, 139, 142, 175, 191, 195, 197, 199, 226, 228, 277
Assignability, 89, 182
attorney, viii, 7, 13, 16, 35, 48, 60, 72, 80, 89, 91, 92, 106, 107, 108, 110, 111, 115, 120, 129, 142, 148, 150, 157, 170, 174, 179, 181, 182, 184, 194, 235, 236, 238, 277

B
Banker, 48
base pay, 195, 206, 207
billing, 107, 122, 124, 135, 156, 209, 210, 222, 224
buy-in, *125, 127, 142, 178, 179, 194*
buy-outs, 125, 290

C
carve out, xi, 91, 181, 283
claims-made, 105
Claims-made, 159
coding, 122, 208, 209
collections, 124, 135, 196, 209, 222, 223, 224
Compensation Models, x, 204
conversion factor, 209, 210, 216

D
deferred compensation, 199
Disability insurance, 198
duties and responsibilities, 175, 176, 177, 251

E
Effect of Termination, 88

F
fair market value, 142, 192, 193, 197, 225, 228, 247, 251

THANK YOU FOR TAKING YOUR VALUABLE TIME TO LEARN HOW TO MAKE THESE CRITICAL POWER MOVES™!

Do not forget to download your personal Power Moves™ Workbook.

"The Doctor's Ultimate Guide to Contracts and Negotiations: Power Moves™ Workbook Plan, Prepare, and Execute"

Download Here:
https://bit.ly/PowerMovesWorkbook

You are also invited to join my Power Moves Book Club today!

Register here:
https://bit.ly/JoinPowerMovesBookClub

#PowerMoves

Made in USA - Crawfordsville, IN
96625_9781513658834
04.20.2023 1804